25p

1

Rheumatism
— What Is It?

This book is about rheumatism. It is about the different kinds of rheumatism and about the ways in which you, a rheumatism sufferer, can help yourself.

Rheumatism is the commonest of all the problems that affect the musculoskeletal system. Most of you will suffer from this complaint at one time or another. Usually the problem is shortlived, but at times it can be prolonged, painful and life-disturbing.

Rheumatism can affect anyone at any age, and can last for days, months or years.

You will find the most effective treatment for rheumatism lies in your own hands. With understanding of the condition and of the skills required to treat it, your problem can be greatly reduced. Your rheumatism can be managed. Your life can become more livable.

The word 'rheumatism' stems from the ancient Greek word *rheumatismos*, which means 'suffering from a flux'.

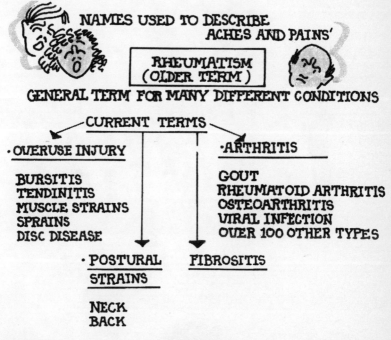

Figure 1

An old word, it was initially used to group a variety of complaints of the musculoskeletal system under the one title (Figure 1). Knowledge of the different types of condition that can cause this 'flux' has grown enormously. We have been able to identify the different types of arthritis and the different types of soft tissue inflammation (i.e. non-bony tissues), all of which can contribute to problems of the body frame.

Today, the term 'rheumatism' continues to be used by many to describe all the aches and pains in the body that don't have special names. It is this group of disorders that this book focuses on.

However, though the word 'rheumatism' continues as a general term, it's possible to classify the types of rheumatism better than ever before. So we will be discussing conditions such as fibrositis, referred pain, chronic pain, and some others. These all come under the rheumatism banner.

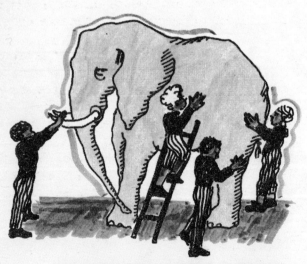

THE BLIND MEN AND THE ELEPHANT
OF RHEUMATISM – LOOK AT WHOLE,
NOT JUST PART OF THE BEAST.

Figure 2

People Who Can Help

The name 'rheumatism' has given rise to the title rheumatologist — a specialist in the study and treatment of rheumatic disorders. These are generally taken as all those afflictions that can affect the musculoskeletal system from arthritis to fibrositis and through to various types of connective tissue disease. So you may go to a rheumatologist to have your arthritis treated. You can also go to a rheumatologist to have your rheumatism treated. But many other people are involved in the management of rheumatism. They include a whole variety of health care professionals: physiotherapists, occupational therapists, chiropractors, osteopaths, exercise specialists, nurses, and a host of others.

Indeed rheumatism is a bit like the old story of the six blind men and the elephant (Figure 2). The elephant is rheumatism, and the six blind men are people who approach this large animal from different angles. Most people see only one part of the elephant and describe it in words they understand, according to the way they were trained.

What this book hopes to do is to look at the *whole elephant* rather than just bits of it. You will then see where the various treatments fit, so that you think of the whole beast, not just one part of it. This will surely lead to better understanding and treatment, and will take the main care of the problem away from the blind men and give it back to the person with the problem. Once people take more responsibility for themselves, the better they will be able to 'manage' their rheumatism.

Arthritis Is Different

Let's leave the topic of rheumatism for a moment, and talk a little about what it is not. Rheumatism is certainly *not arthritis*. Arthritis relates to disease or damage in a joint. There are over 100 different types of arthritis, but most of them fall into two categories: *inflammation* and *degeneration.* Examples of inflammatory arthritis include gout, rheumatoid arthritis, and psoriatic arthritis (remember the curious case of *The Singing Detective*!). Osteoarthritis and arthritis after injury to a joint are examples of degenerative arthritis.

Figure 3 shows a typical joint. The synovial membrane lines the inner part of the joint and produces fluid for lubrication and nutrition of the joint surfaces. They are composed of joint cartilage.

Inflammation in a joint usually affects the synovial membrane (Figure 4), and extra fluid is produced. This causes the joint to swell. The fluid so produced contains many chemicals which, among other things, irritate the pain nerves lining the joint. So inflammatory arthritis is often very painful.

If arthritis occurs quickly, it is called *acute.* Gout is a typical example of acute inflammatory arthritis. Where arthritis has a slower onset and lasts longer, it is called *chronic* arthritis. Rheumatoid arthritis is such an example.

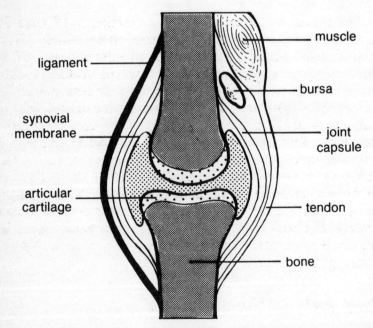

Figure 3 *Normal joint*

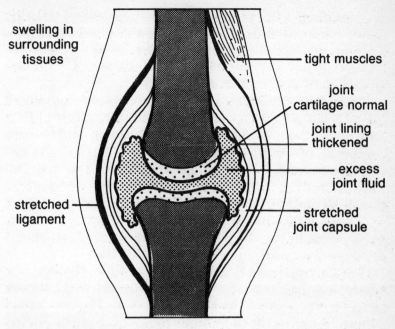

swelling in surrounding tissues

tight muscles

joint cartilage normal

joint lining thickened

excess joint fluid

stretched ligament

stretched joint capsule

Figure 4 *Inflamed joint*

Degenerative arthritis, e.g. osteoarthritis (Figure 5), has to do with the intactness of the joint cartilage. Normal shiny healthy cartilage starts to deteriorate, often for unknown reasons. The joint surfaces become roughened. Mild inflammation of the synovial membrane with swelling in the joints may occur, but the main brunt of the injury and damage occurs to the cartilage. Eventually deformity and pain are possible. This type of arthritis is more insidious than inflammatory arthritis, and often takes years before you feel any symptoms. Indeed x-rays will show signs of mild to moderate osteoarthritis in most people, particularly as you age; yet, as a rule, few people ever suffer any symptoms as a consequence. In other words degenerative arthritis is usually without symptoms, at least early in its life.

Arthritis Is Well Defined

The various kinds of arthritis have been studied for

many years. They are well defined for classification, progress and treatment. Though the causes of most types of arthritis are unknown, they are all a bit different from each other and they all have specific names. These conditions then are *not* rheumatism.

Other musculoskeletal tissues can become inflamed. Figure 6 shows these. Sometimes physical stress can be the cause. Sometimes it's a disease process which focuses on the synovial membrane such as with rheumatoid arthritis or gout.

The synovial membrane that lines the inner joint is also present in other parts of the body. When this tissue is between a bone and a muscle or between two muscles, it is called a *bursa*. The bursa forms a little sac of enclosed fluid that allows tissues like this to run over each other in a smooth way. Bursae allow the body to move smoothly by lubricating the 'rough bits'. There are many bursae around the shoulder, hip and knees in particular. In fact in the body as a whole, there are hundreds of bursae. If there's excessive strain on the bursa, the

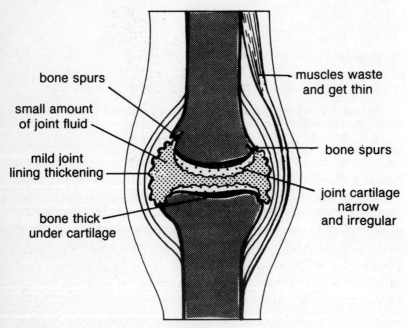

Figure 5 *Degenerative arthritis*

thin membrane becomes inflamed and produces extra
fluid. That fluid contains many painful substances, and
the diagnosis is *bursitis*. The exact type of bursitis
depends on where the bursa is situated. Trochanteric
bursitis is a typical example. Here the bursa sitting
between the outer side of the bone of the upper thigh and
the overlying muscles gets inflamed, and the area
becomes exquisitely tender and sore. This is one of the
causes of hip pain.

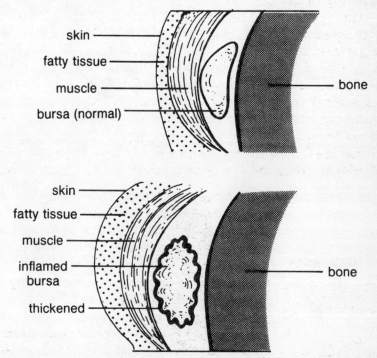

skin
fatty tissue
muscle
bursa (normal)
bone

skin
fatty tissue
muscle
inflamed
bursa
thickened
bone

Figure 6 *Bursa (e.g. over the bone) before and after inflammation*

A similar membrane lines tendons — particularly
where they run through small tunnels or over areas that
need smooth friction-free movement of the tendon. Take
the tendon pulleys of the hand or the tendons around the
ankle or wrist. If the membrane gets inflamed in these
areas, it is called *tenosynovitis* (Figure 7). This will also
produce swelling and pain. Because the tendons are so
crucial to the function of say the hand, you will notice

some loss of that function and a developing stiffness. So inflammation of these membranes leads to pain, stiffness, swelling and loss of use.

Some other important musculoskeletal tissues are not lined by synovial membrane, but they can still become

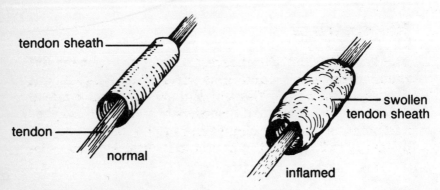

tendon (in sheath) before and after inflammation

Figure 7 *Tenosynovitis*

inflamed due to excessive movement, local injury or an underlying disease process. The tissues between the junction of muscle and tendon and the bone to which the tendon attaches are very prone to this kind of problem (Figure 8).

Tennis elbow is a good example. Forceful movement of forearm and hand may pull on the sensitive tissues around the elbow. There the muscles form into a tendon and the tendon attaches to the bone. (This goes under the technical name of *enthesitis* because enthesis is the name for the tissue which attaches to bone.) If the inflammation is in other structures (e.g. a ligament or tendon), then it is called *ligamentitis* or *tendinitis*. These problems occur often around the shoulder: the capsule of this joint becomes inflamed, giving rise to *capsulitis*.

Nerves may be squeezed or pressured by bones or discs moving out of their normal position. This will cause sudden severe pain, often with a change in sensation. These conditions are well defined and usually easily diagnosed. They are not rheumatism.

Muscles may also become strained or torn, and again these types of problems have specific names and treatments. You are all familiar with muscle pain or aching (called *myalgia*), particularly after doing heavy work or sport. These are the normal aches and pains of everyday living.

Rheumatism

You have just read about several conditions that are not rheumatism. Those conditions affect either joints or soft tissues (i.e. non-bony tissues). But rheumatism is indeed different. It is a group of disorders that can cause aches and pains, stiffness or change in function of the body. It primarily relates to the musculoskeletal system. The

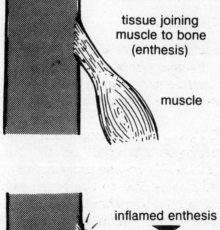

tissue joining
muscle to bone
(enthesis)

muscle

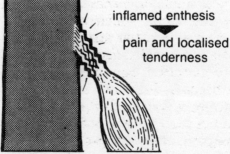

inflamed enthesis

pain and localised
tenderness

Figure 8 *Inflammation of tendon bone junction (e.g. tennis elbow)*

type of rheumatism that is most troublesome is the chronic or recurring type. There's less to worry about with acute or sudden pain in the neck or back that settles quite quickly with rest or other management. Ongoing problems are a bigger concern — that is, those which lead you to wonder what is the cause of the pain and what to do about it. After all, pain *is* the main symptom of rheumatism. Its companions are stiffness, fatigue and change in function. To begin our understanding of rheumatism, let's look a bit at pain.

2

Pain and Rheumatism

In this chapter, the focus is on two types of pain. The first is caused by a stimulus near the surface of the body, so-called *superficial pain*. Then there's pain due to stimulation of tissues deep within the body, so-called *deep pain*.

Superficial Pain

Pricking the finger with a needle is superficial pain. In this case the pain comes quickly after the needle prick. It is sharp and local, reaches a peak quickly, and dies off quickly. You may be left with a dull ache for several minutes afterwards, and the spot will be tender for a day or so. Usually little else occurs.

● Well, what happens here? Firstly, the point of the needle breaks through the skin. It excites fine nerve fibres under the surface of the skin. The nerve fibres which record pain are plentiful, but are more concentrated in some areas than in others. They are plentiful in the skin of the hand and other sensitive spots, but are

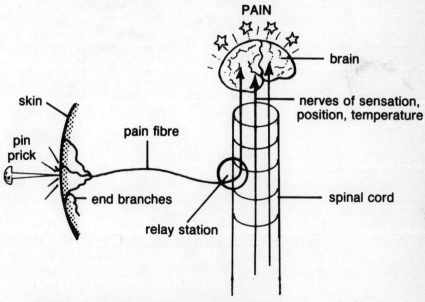

Figure 1 *Pain nerve joining spinal cord*

fewer in the trunk of the body. A fine pain nerve fibre is thinner than a cotton thread; and because these pain nerves are so small, it has been difficult to study them closely until recently.

When the nerve is stimulated, a message is transmitted along the nerve fibre to the spinal cord (Figure 1). The spinal cord is a collection of nerve fibres which carry nerve messages relating to many functions, not just the recording of pain. This group of fibres makes a large bundle or cord of nerve fibres and connects with the brain. The pain nerves send their message to the spinal cord, and a pain relay station sits at the entrance to the spinal cord (Figure 2). In the relay station there are many other nerve fibres, not just pain nerve fibres. For instance, impulses and messages come from muscles in the same area as that which the pain nerve serves. Impulses also come from the sensation nerves in the skin around

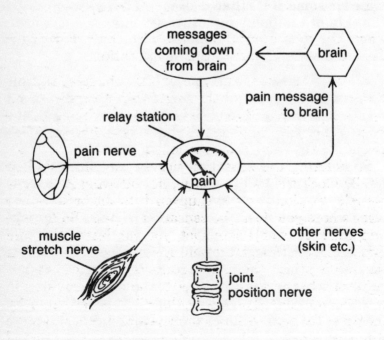

Figure 2 *Pain relay station*

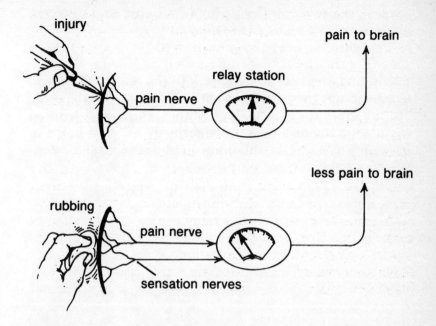

Figure 3 *Skin sensation nerves block pain at relay station*

where the pain occurs. Impulses also come down from
the brain and connect to this relay station.

● The pain message may never leave the relay station.
For instance, a prick of the finger with a needle, or hit
with a hammer, will lead to instinctive rubbing of the
finger. This will stimulate the nerves of sensation, which
also go to the same relay station (Figure 3).
Stimulating the sensation nerves can often dull or
totally block the pain message, not allowing it to leave
the relay station and travel upwards to the brain — the
place where you 'feel' the sensation of pain. So by rubbing the area over a sore spot, you can lessen the pain
message. Even though the pain stimulus continues (from
the needle prick), the pain *message* is blocked by stimulation of other nerves connected to the same relay station
in the spinal cord. By the way, this effect is used in many
therapies for pain — for example, transcutaneous nerve
stimulation in which the sensation nerves are stimulated
by electrical impulses, in an effort to block the pain mes-

sage at the relay station. Simple rubbing and massage will often have a similar result.

The muscles near the pain nerve also have a role to play (Figure 4). Stimulating those muscles and the connecting nerve fibres that go back to the relay station will again disrupt the pain message — blocking it at the relay station. Pain from arms, for instance, can be interrupted by moving the arm muscles vigorously. All this helps to explain why exercise and movement are so vital for people who have chronic pain.

● Most important of all, the third influence on the relay station is the brain. This is marvellously demon-

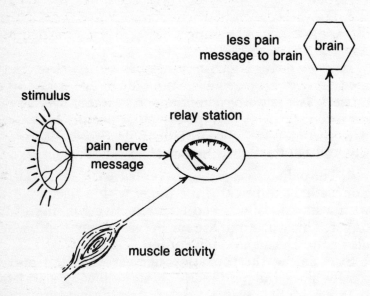

Figure 4 *Increasing muscle activity decreases pain message at relay station*

strated by yogis who, through meditation, can so train their higher nervous system (and its influences on the relay station) that they can block the pain message right out. After lots of training, yogis can sit on nails for long periods, showing no discomfort whatsoever. Yet each single nail is stimulating the pain nerve system constantly.

Once again, the pain is simply blocked out at the relay station. It does not get a chance to come up to the higher centres.

Pain, then, always includes a psychological response. As you move through life, you learn to link various psychological reactions with pain. A simple example is lining up for an inoculation needle at school. Some people don't bat an eyelid.They feel a shortlived jab of discomfort and pass on to the next event in life. Others worry a lot beforehand, perhaps sweating or shaking or even fainting — all this before the needle jab!

Everyone is anxious to some degree when faced with pain. Have you ever gripped the arm of a dentist's chair, even before he has started the procedure? You are also familiar with the child who is screaming with pain. Simple comforting and 'kissing it better' usually dull the pain and end the distress.

How we deal with pain influences our reaction to the next set of painful stimuli. Pain may be accompanied by anxiety, fear, or other emotions. It is sometimes used to get attention or to manipulate other people. It is a very powerful weapon in family situations. So it's just impossible to separate psychological events from the pain

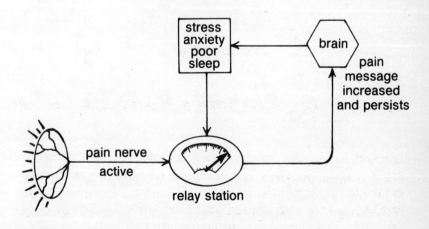

Figure 5 *Emotional factors amplify pain message*

itself. Some people worry about the possible psychological or emotional effects of their reaction to pain.
However, pain is a fact of life, and part of the pain is how
your mind and emotions deal with it (Figure 5).

Substance P Is Released

Now, let's go back to the needle prick in the skin. When
the needle stimulates a pain nerve, a small hormone,
called substance P, is released. This small hormone is
made within the nerve and is mainly found at nerve ends.
When substance P is released (after a traumatic event or
an injury), then the hormone will have other effects on
the surrounding tissues. Substance P, when released into
these tissues, causes fluid to flow from the blood vessels
into the tissues. This partly produces the swelling that
accompanies an injury. It also increases the blood supply

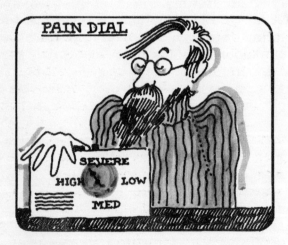

Figure 6

into the area, and the skin around the injury reddens.
This is known by the technical term *dermatographia*, or
the 'red reaction'.

In some cases, although the pain stimulus may be
shortlived, the pain message lasts. This is particularly so
when the relay station is faulty. The main problem here

is with the messages coming downward from the brain. Here, due to poorly understood central factors such as psychological or emotional events, the pain message is not blocked off and passes through the relay station very easily. Indeed the pain may become worse and persist. Think of this like turning up the volume of your radio. The radio is the pain sensation, the dial the relay station. Though the needle has left the skin a long time before, the tissues continue to send the pain message. We don't know the cause of this persisting pain. Indeed it's the basic problem for most people with chronic pain and other lasting rheumatism problems. However, it seems that change in the brain's downward messages is important, and this particularly links with psychological events in our lives (Figure 6).

Deep Pain

When you have pain from deep tissues, a similar series of events occurs, but there are other important things to note. Pain deep in the tissues does not tell you much about where it is located in the body — not like the very local pain from a pin prick. You may sense some pain as achy or burning rather than sharp like the pin prick. But pain from deep stimulation often lasts a lot longer, and aches for several hours or days after the pain stimulus has stopped. Deep pain sensation is carried along the same fine nerve fibres and uses the same substance P hormone mechanism as before. The sensation goes to the relay station in the spine and similar influences occur on its message. However, the pain nerve fibres also interact with other important structures in the relay centre (Figure 7).

● Firstly, there is interaction with muscle fibres. Deep pain *automatically* causes stimulation of the muscle fibres around it. The muscle tightens. In fact, muscle tightness can be more uncomfortable than the pain which caused it. This is more so when anxiety or other emotional factors add to muscle tightness.

● Secondly, deep pain activates skin blood vessels more dramatically than superficial pain, and reddening and swelling occur.

● Thirdly, as we have noted, pain from deep down is not local, but spread over a wider area of the body. This is called *referred pain.*
Because the stimulated part is deep within the body, it is difficult for you to feel or know where it starts. For instance, on a day-to-day basis, you have no idea where your appendix or gall bladder or stomach is. If one of these becomes painful, the pain message is sent to the surface of the body. This is because, at the relay station, pain fibres and sensation fibres come together.The pain fibres stir up the sensation fibres. Appendicitis gives achy pain around the belly button, and only later does pain occur over the true appendix position in the right lower abdomen.

Take another example of referred pain. If the gall bladder is inflamed, pain is often felt low on the right-hand side of the chest. In this case, the sensation fibres and the gall bladder pain fibres meet up in the spinal cord.

Reflex Changes

These sorts of changes are called reflex changes. In other words, stimulating pain nerves in one area will, reflexly and automatically, activate other nerves and set off other events in the body. Muscle tightness, skin reaction and swelling, and referred pain on the surface of the body are examples of reflex changes. Other reflex changes from deep pain include changes in some other organs of the body, e.g. the stomach or bowel. For instance, pain that begins in the abdominal muscles may cause nausea and vomiting.

We have not yet discussed one of the most important reflex changes. This is when there is tenderness in tissues well away from the source of the deep pain. It is hard to believe at first and causes some confusion. An interesting experiment has been tried. If an irritating amount of salt solution is injected into the deep ligaments of the back, then all the different qualities of deep pain will emerge. These occur *without* any involvement of the large nerve which might cause sciatica. You will find that pain is distributed in a predictable pattern, depending on which spinal ligament is stimulated. The muscles in the

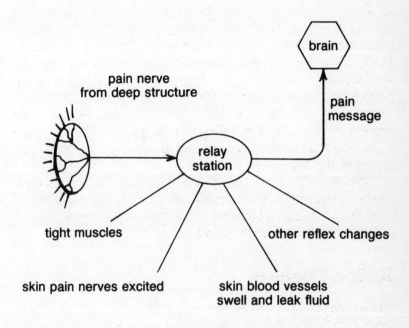

Figure 7 *Pain from deep structures automatically activates other nerves*

area start to tighten, and the skin changes colour and reacts differently to stimuli. Importantly, some spots nearby become tender, as do others further away from the pain. We can show this by one example: have a look at Figure 8.

Every level of the spine stimulated like this has a different but predictable pattern. So tenderness in the fatty tissues around the knee may be caused by a stimulus deep in the low back; indeed this is a common event.

Tenderness in the soft tissues around the buttock can be caused by low back problems, and tenderness just below the elbow can be due to deep neck problems. These tender spots are well known and have been confirmed in experiments. They are often not recognised by the person with the pain until discovered by examination.

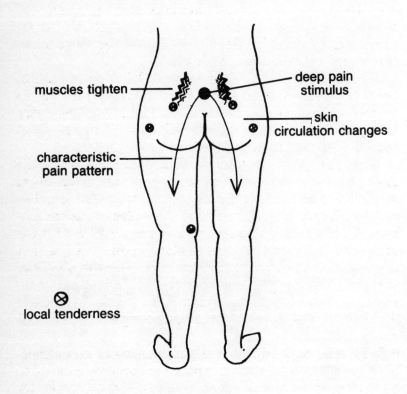

Figure 8 *Tenderness occurs in tissues away from deep pain source*

Control System and Deep Pain

Now, what about the control system and its tie with deep pain? If the relay station is faulty, the consequences for deep pain may be dramatic. Suppose the deep pain message reaches the relay station and does not have the normal amount of inhibition from the brain's circuitry, which includes psychological effects. You will then have greater pain. The increased pain will activate all the reflexes we have been discussing. So there will be even more marked referred pain, tender points, muscle tightness, and skin circulation changes. The effects on the viscera — i.e. the stomach, the bowel, other organs — may also be marked. Local pain gets built up because all the pain pathways and reflexes which relate to the initiating deep stimulus have been amplified. More about this when we talk about fibrositis.

A heart attack is a vivid example of deep pain. The heart lies deep within the chest. If a small artery on the surface of the heart is blocked, blood will not get to the heart muscle and the muscle will die. The amount of muscle involved is about the size of a small coin.

With change in the muscle comes stimulation of the pain nerves, and this deep pain may show up in other ways. The person has a funny feeling in the left hand — maybe a heavy feeling or pins and needles or just numbness. There is less strength in the grip. Further up the arm, there's a sense of a breeze blowing on it, as if a door is open in the room. Further up still, over the shoulder and the chest, the pain is crushing. All these pain sensations come from the same little piece of muscle involved in the heart attack, but not everyone experiences them all.

The sensations of referred pain are many and varied, but they are well known. The pain may be severe for up to an hour or more, but the chest wall and arm may ache for hours or even days. The pain is accompanied by muscle tightening particularly around the chest wall and arm, and circulation changes can be recorded on the surface of the skin of the upper chest wall — particularly on the left side. The person may vomit. There may be sweating and other changes in the body. Anyone who has a relative who has had angina or a heart attack will find that these characteristics are fairly common. Such are the qualities of deep pain.

Well then, how does all this relate to rheumatism? In
fact, most of the features of deep pain are the same as
those of rheumatism. In a nutshell, you may say that
activation of the pain system — especially when the pain
comes from deep down — will give rise to the many
symptoms typical of rheumatic pain. These symptoms
may be shortlived or lasting. Lasting symptoms may
have to do with other influences in the spine that alter
and amplify the message to the brain. These secondary
reflexes have their own sets of symptoms — e.g. stiffness,
discomfort and swelling. Knowing these things helps us
to devise ways of coping with rheumatic pain that are not
obvious at the start.

3

Neck Pain

Neck pain is very common. Almost every day, you experience pain or discomfort in the neck. Luckily, most times neck pain is mild and passes away quickly. The cause is usually obvious, and simple measures prevent it coming back. However, at other times neck pain is severe and lasts for a long time. Chronic neck pain, for example, is most distressing.

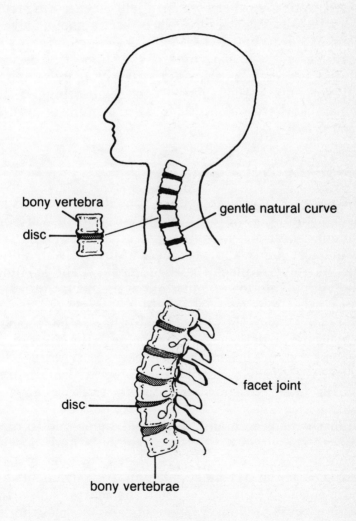

Figure 1 *Simple anatomy of the neck*

In this chapter let's focus on chronic neck pain, what causes it and how to treat it. Most people with bad neck pain can be taught to help themselves.

What's better than to start at the beginning! The neck supports the head in the erect posture. The head itself weighs 4.5 kg (about ten pounds). This weight is propped up by the bony structure of the neck, the cervical vertebrae. There are seven of these vertebrae. Each is separated from the other by a firm jelly encased in strong fibre. This is called a disc. Each disc is about half the width of a vertebra, so cervical discs contribute to your height as well as the strength of the supporting cervical column. The head is then supported by bony vertebrae and soft discs that give a shock-absorbing effect. Remember there is a natural forward bending of the neck (Figure 1).

What the Neck Can Do

The neck is able to move in various directions and has special joints at the back of the supporting vertebral column. These special joints are called *facet joints*. The lower facet joints allow the neck to move from side to side, letting you place the ear almost on the shoulder. The middle and lower joints allow the neck to turn, so that you can look over your shoulder to right or left. The upper joints, with the help of some others, allow the neck to bend forward; the chin can drop onto the chest or the neck be extended back so you can see upwards. The movements of the neck are highly integrated, and a problem in one part of it will often cause change in another.

For the neck to maintain normal shape and to move around, there are supporting ligaments and muscles. There are many levels of these. Deep down against the bone, you will find strong tight supporting ligaments and short muscles. Further out from the central supporting column, there are longer ligaments and muscles that restrain the neck like a circus tent or pull it in certain directions.

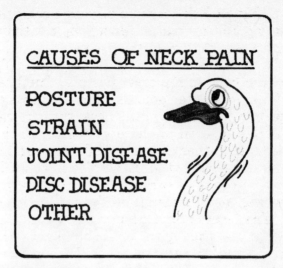

CAUSES OF NECK PAIN

POSTURE
STRAIN
JOINT DISEASE
DISC DISEASE
OTHER

Figure 2

There is a tube between the back of the supporting vertebral column and the place where the joints are located. This tube is a tunnel for the nerves going in and out of the brain. Smaller nerves branch off from this large spinal nerve bundle (or cord) and pass out of other small holes called the *intervertebral foramen*. These holes form very close to the facet joints. Joint abnormalities can thus pinch nerves travelling from the spine to the arm.

Neck pain occurs for several reasons (Figure 2). The most common cause by far is strain or unusual tension on the supporting ligaments and joint-lining structures in the lower neck. Another possible reason is arthritis of the facet joints. The most common is a form of osteoarthritis, but rheumatoid arthritis, and occasionally other types of arthritis, can also affect these joints.

The disc may also be a source of neck pain. If the disc's supporting membrane is weak, the disc may bulge and press onto a nerve. This process irritates the nerve and causes symptoms of nerve root irritation and compression. Taken all together, these causes account for over 98% of neck pain.

Young Necks

Let's assume there's neck pain, yet no disease in the disc or facet joint. A common enough situation. Here neck pain may be acute or chronic. The acute situation is the one you have all experienced. You awaken in the morning with a tight, stiff and sore neck. It's usually painful low on one side of the neck, and more to the back than the

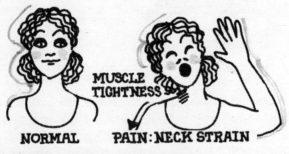

SUDDEN ONSET OF NECK PAIN

Figure 3

front. To move the neck just a little is very sore. It's an aching pain, usually fairly local. However, you may find the aching goes up into the muscles at the back of your neck, or aching pain radiates between the shoulder blades or across the trapezius muscle (the main muscle of the upper back) to the shoulder. At other times the pain radiates into the arm itself. This is the so-called 'wry neck' or *acute torticollis* (Figure 3). The cause of this problem has much to do with posture, as do many of the neck's problems.

Night-time posture of a neck is extremely important. You spend about eight hours of each twenty-four lying on your side or back, the neck often in an unsupported position. The head, shoulder and back may be supported, but the middle of the neck is often neglected (Figure 4). This puts great strain on the neck; and at times, during a heavy sleep in an abnormal position, one of the structures deep in the neck gets overstretched or strained. It's

SLEEP POSTURE AND THE NECK

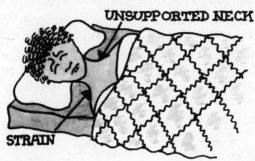

UNSUPPORTED NECK

STRAIN

Figure 4

usually the ligaments or the joint capsules that are involved. They are very sensitive to pain. To stretch them abnormally stirs up the pain nerves which are part of the ligaments or joint capsules. Pain nerves, activated so, may reflexly tighten surrounding muscles.

Besides this, there are other nerve endings in these structures. They are called *mechanoreceptors*. They respond to mechanical stretch, and big stretches will activate these nerves. In turn, once these nerve endings are stimulated beyond a certain point, other structures get reflexly activated.

The main structures so excited are again the muscles around the ligamentous stretch. So deep ligament stretch activates muscles in their own right, independent of the pain pathway. This results in stiffness and sometimes muscle spasm, bringing on its own set of painful symptoms. Worse pain can occur just through these ligament-nerve-muscle pathways (Figure 5).

We have already discussed the consequences of deep pain. If the pain is deep in the neck, then it may also be felt in other predictable locations some way from the neck. So head pain, chest pain, shoulder pain, and arm and hand pain may all link with neck problems. Tender spots may occur in the shoulder, elbow and in the soft tissues between thumb and first finger. This is part of the deep pain reflex activation of other nerves which we talked about before.

Other Reflex Sensations

Pain coming from deep in the neck, e.g. a strained ligament, brings on other reflex sensations. It's very common to feel numbness or pins and needles in the hands
when the neck is the culprit. This tingling is part of referred pain. It is not due to irritation or damage of the
large nerves leaving the spinal cord through the intervertebral passage. This is a very important point. Such
symptoms are often explained on the basis of a 'pinched
nerve' by some therapists. This is not true. These sensations are automatic reflexes.

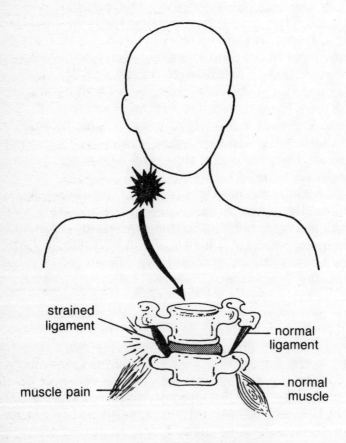

Figure 5 *Muscle pain caused by ligament strain*

Another sensation felt as a consequence of deep pain in the neck is swelling of the hands. This is common in the mornings particularly. It usually recedes through the day.

People who develop sudden acute neck strain usually have neck pain and stiffness as their main problem. Those with longer standing, or chronic, neck strain have less pain in the neck. Instead they may have aching and tightness, particularly when moving the neck in one direction, or some of those abnormal feelings in the arms.

Sue was 28, married and had two children. She complained of pins and needles in her right hand and a sensation of swelling in the hand in the morning. Her elbow and shoulder ached. She had some tightness in the neck. This had been the case for several weeks, and she could think of no obvious cause for it.

Examination showed that Sue's major nerves were working normally and all the muscles contracting normally. What was abnormal, however, was some tenderness in her neck, especially on the right lower side. Her symptoms were in fact due to deep neck pain from soft tissue strain, with pain and other sensations referred into the arm. When this was understood, her symptoms could be tackled.

Older Necks

As we age, it's usual to find changes in the tissues both of the supporting part of the neck and the movable part of the neck. The most common stresses and strains occur low in the neck. Over time, changes occur both in discs (with discs narrowing due to loss of water content), and in the facet joints where cartilage changes occur that lead to osteoarthritis. In some people structural changes in discs or joints will stir up pain nerves. For instance, if the facet joint becomes osteoarthritic, then the structure of that joint changes. The cartilage surfaces are narrowed and bone grows at the edges of the joint. The joint does not move as well, and as we age it's harder to bend the neck to the side. The joint becomes more prone to minor injury; it is just not as supple as it was earlier in life. So the facet joints are more easily sprained or jarred by routine activities.

● People with osteoarthritis in the small joints of the neck are much more prone to routine stresses and strains on the neck in everyday life. Besides the extra risk of

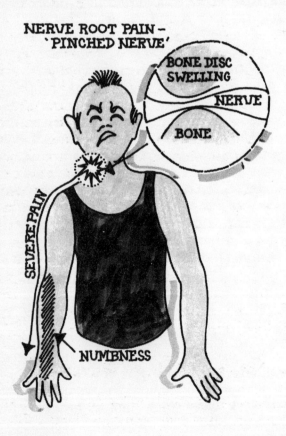

Figure 6

strain, the joint may show symptoms of arthritis itself. This process usually goes through cycles. Inflammation in the joint may cause increased pain, yet later the whole situation will settle again.

● Another problem in the arthritic neck is caused by the bone that grows at the edge of the arthritic joint. The bone can start to close off the intervertebral foramen through which the large nerves pass. At times the larger nerves are pinched as a longterm result of osteoarthritis of the joints. The discs narrow and bulge into the space, causing further narrowing of the canal. Also, when the disc has narrowed, the two vertebral bodies come closer. Extra strain is put on the joint at the back, and there is further osteoarthritic deterioration in the facet joints.

The symptoms that arise from all this are similar to those of the young neck. Deep pain in the neck may be local or radiate out in the same way as with deep referred pain. One major difference occurs if a nerve is pinched (Figure 6). In this situation more severe and well defined pain occurs. The pain shoots down the arm, often linked with tingling or change in muscle function in a specific way that is easily localised by examination. This is quite different to the tingling and numbness which occurs as part of referred pain. These two types of nerve sensation are easily differentiated. One is due to large nerve irritation, the less common situation. The other is due to activation of the very fine pain nerves, the more common situation.

Even though the older neck can give a double helping of trouble (i.e. problems from routine deep strains and problems from 'wear and tear' osteoarthritis), neck pain is luckily not a necessary part of ageing. Most episodes can be helped, and chronic pain lessened.

Tension Makes Things Worse

Increased nervous tension makes deep pain in the neck worse. Tension takes two pathways (Figure 7).

● Firstly, if you are under lots of stress or strain, your

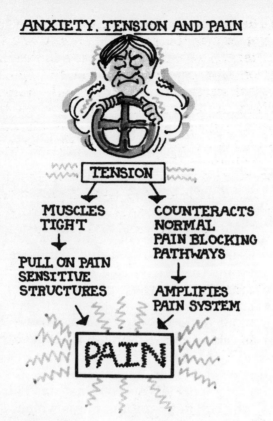

ANXIETY, TENSION AND PAIN

TENSION

MUSCLES
TIGHT
↓
PULL ON PAIN
SENSITIVE
STRUCTURES

COUNTERACTS
NORMAL
PAIN BLOCKING
PATHWAYS
↓
AMPLIFIES
PAIN SYSTEM

PAIN

Figure 7

muscles begin to tighten. Any pain in the neck tends to
magnify, as the tight muscles pull pain-sensitive structures together. Muscle tension is well known. It occurs
when you drive in heavy traffic. It occurs after a hard
day's work. It occurs if you worry a lot about life's problems. The muscles of the neck are just so sensitive to
everday tension. You must *always* consider tight muscles
as a possible cause of pain in the neck. It's very typical for
a simple neck strain to occur through, for instance, poor
sleep posture. A strained ligament deep in the neck
results in pain made worse by tense muscles. Relief of
tension will usually allow simple treatment to help the
underlying ligamentous strain problem. If the tension is
not fixed, the strain may persist and get worse, and
chronic vicious cycles can occur.

● The second way tension aggravates neck pain is as follows. Remember the pain system and the fact that pain is influenced by pathways between the brain and the relay station (for pain sensation at the spinal cord). Psychological stress and tension greatly influence the pain received into the central nervous system. If you are under a lot of psychological stress, then pain sensation gets greater, not less, because of the change in these so important control pathways.

So tight muscles pull on pain-sensitive structures and increase pain. In addition, the psychological tension that causes tight muscles will amplify pain pathways, further activate deep pain reflexes, and make the situation much worse.

Some Ways to Help

Neck pain is all too familiar. You have usually experienced it in the not too distant past and know ways to cope

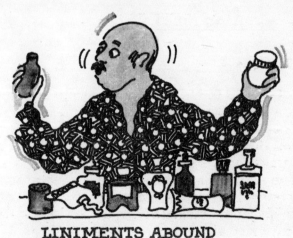

LINIMENTS ABOUND

Figure 8

with it. It may be that you ignore it, go through the day as usual, and let the situation run its course over the next few days. If you need quicker relief, there is some definite action that can be taken.

● Heat is useful. A hot water bottle wrapped in a towel and applied to the painful area will ease the pain and often relax the tight muscles aggravating the problem. Heat can be used indefinitely while the pain is present. There is a sackful of commonly purchased liniments which also heat the tissues. The massage used when liniments are applied also helps sore muscles (Figure 8).

● Think too about your working environment. Maybe a work posture does not suit you. Perhaps it's an awkward or prolonged posture, and you need a change in the way you work or in your posture (Figure 9). A change to your chair or desk, or in the order of your jobs, often does the trick.

● More likely, though, the problem comes from bad sleep posture. You must have good support to the neck, particularly while pain persists. The pillow should be a single shallow pillow supporting the neck as much as the head (Figure 10). Sleeping on the back or the side is all

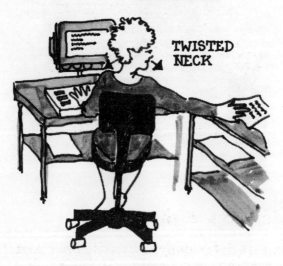

WORK POSTURE AND NECK PAIN

TWISTED NECK

Figure 9

right, but not on the stomach with the neck twisted to the side.

● Simple painkillers may be needed. Medication such as soluble aspirin, one or two taken every four hours, can give quick relief. Paracetamol, one or two four hourly, is a suitable alternative for some. If muscle spasm is a major part of the problem, then occasionally medication aimed at muscle spasm may be given by your doctor.

● If the problem is severe or not settling quickly, physical treatment can help. Physiotherapists use various pieces of equipment to place heat deep into the tissues. These include the use of ultrasound and interferential. Gentle movement or manipulation of one or several spinal segments helps free up a set of spinal segments tightened by muscle constriction (Figure 11). In this case, there is no partial subluxation or full dislocation of the neck. The structures of the neck are in normal alignment. The neck is not 'out'. The muscles have merely tightened, squashing the joints and other pain-sensitive structures close together and leading to persistent pain in that area.

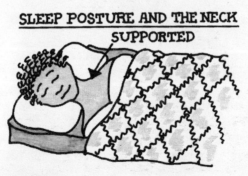

SLEEP POSTURE AND THE NECK
SUPPORTED

Figure 10

Chronic Pain in the Neck

The same principles apply to chronic neck pain. Look at the posture of the neck. Low-grade abnormalities in posture are the key to symptoms in chronic neck pain.

Again, night-time posture needs to be checked. There may be a case for support in the form of a cervical neck ruff. It's a simple piece of equipment you can make at home or with a health professional's help. The idea is to increase support for the nape of the neck and minimise any shearing forces that continually stress the joints and ligaments giving the symptoms. Such supports are really mini-pillows. The one shown here costs very little to make. The outer part can be washed regularly, and the

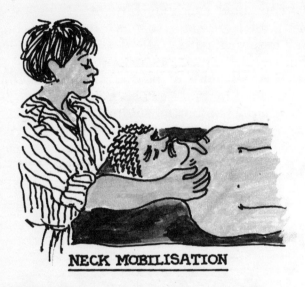

NECK MOBILISATION

Figure 11

inner cotton wool replaced at minimal cost (Figure 12). Cervical ruffs are simple, practical, and usually work well. They are tied loosely around the front of the neck so that you don't roll off the support in the night. Other more complicated pillows and supports are available, but they cost a lot more. Don't buy such a pillow until you try the simple approach first.

With chronic neck pain, it's sensible to think of therapy to help loosen the tight segments in the low neck. A physical therapist first concentrates on gradual loosening of the tissues through heat or more sophisticated devices. Then gentle hand-directed movements loosen the neck (i.e. mobilisation). Sometimes manipulation, a more forceful movement, will achieve results quicker. Before manipulation, the therapist makes sure there is no underlying structural damage to the neck and the diagnosis is correct. Different therapists, even if trained in the same field, will often have an individual approach to an identical problem. So it's clear that different physical approaches will achieve the same result — loosening of the neck and loss of the pain.

Exercises are very much to be encouraged. Important

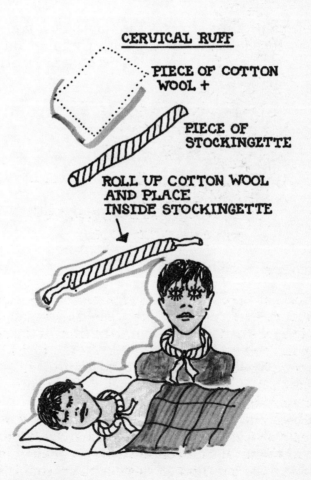

CERVICAL RUFF

PIECE OF COTTON WOOL +

PIECE OF STOCKINGETTE

ROLL UP COTTON WOOL AND PLACE INSIDE STOCKINGETTE

Figure 12

ones are those for rotation of the neck and stretching tight areas in the neck. These will be discussed in some detail later.

As with acute pain, medication may be necessary. However, it should be kept as simple as possible. If neck pain and other symptoms are disabling, more powerful medication can be used. But at no time are narcotic medications, e.g. morphine, pethidine, or codeine, ever given for chronic soft-tissue neck pain.

Evaluate Your Stresses

Aside from posture, stress is the single most important thing to consider. The person with chronic pain must carefully evaluate the stresses in his or her life. Stresses

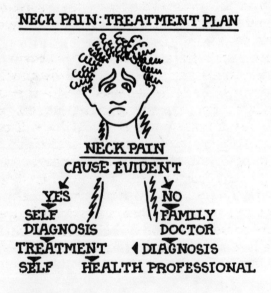

Figure 13

may be hidden or even denied. But they are usually there. Of course, what is stress to one person may not be perceived as stress to another. Each of us has a very personal stress profile. Stress and its relationship to neck pain are so critical that they are discussed further in a later chapter that gives specific suggestions on the management of stress.

If neck pain is due to osteoarthritis, then medication may be helpful for the inflammatory component. Your family doctor may prescribe one of the common anti-inflammatory medications. They are useful: they are generally long-acting and often only one or two doses each day are enough. They are also very effective, and in 95% of people are free of significant side-effects. Stomach upsets with anti-inflammatory medication are more likely in tense people, often giving a clue to underlying stress. Taken as a whole, though, they are a very safe group of medications.

The osteoarthritic neck must be treated much more gently than the normal neck. So take care in choosing the right physical therapist. Ask around or get advice from your doctor. It is far better for the situation to be reviewed by a doctor before you start out on some physical treatment.

An outline for managing neck pain is shown in Figure 13. The key is to begin with a good diagnosis. Many simple pains can be self-diagnosed. But if they are more severe or last longer than usual, then involve your local family doctor. Sometimes further advice will be sought from specialists. Once the diagnosis is obtained, then the treatment plan can begin. But remember that most treatments for common neck pains can be done by the person with the problem, without outside help. Yet it is important not to ignore that many healthcare professionals are extremely good at helping neck pain. Sometimes the best way is team effort between the therapist and yourself.

Resistant Problems

Some people with neck pain will have tried all these techniques, yet their pain continues. It is unfortunately true that some situations are harder to treat than others, but most should settle or improve significantly using the above plan. If neck pain resists standard treatment, then it's essential to check the diagnosis is correct. More discussion, examination and sometimes more elaborate investigation are needed.

One of the common reasons for persistent neck pain is the development of localised fibrositis. This just means that the pain-nerve system is more active and becomes self-perpetuating. This is not so for the patient with simple neck pain and some routine excitement of the pain system. Special approaches are needed in this case, and they are taken up later.

4

Low Back
Pain

Rheumatic pain in the low back happens spontaneously, or it can follow an injury or a degenerative process to one of the parts of the lumbar spine. Before we consider the different causes of back pain, let's look at the structure and function of the low back or lumbar region.

There are five lumbar vertebrae, each separated from the other by a lumbar vertebral disc (Figure 1). The disc

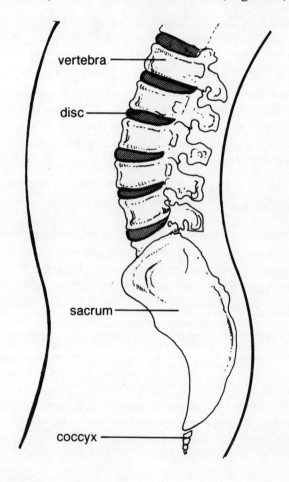

Figure 1 *Lumbar spine*

is one third of the height of the vertebra. Taken together the vertebral bodies (which are made of bone) and the discs (which are made of gelatinous material) support the weight of your body. The discs cushion you during movement and action of the low back. The lumbar spine has a natural curve, much like the shape of the banana. The curve is gentle and is termed *lordosis*. Some people are born with a greater curve in the lumbar spine than others — this condition is called hyperlordosis or increased lordosis — and gives rise to the descriptive term 'sway back'.

The main function of the lumbar spine is to carry the weight of the body. The lumbar spine will bend forward and straighten, but it does not go beyond that. It will also arch back a little, but not greatly. The mechanics of the lumbar spine create enormous pressure and torque forces on the lowest parts of the lumbar spine. This is particularly so in the area between the 5th lumbar vertebra and the sacrum, on which the lumbar spine rests and connects through another disc.

High Rate of Degeneration

With age, increased stress in the lowermost part of the spine leads to a high rate of degeneration of the disc in the same part of the spine. The most common disc to deteriorate is indeed the disc between the 5th lumbar vertebra and the sacrum, the so-called L5-S1 disc. This disc may not just degenerate slowly; it may also rupture beyond its normal confines, spilling some of its gelatinous material into the surrounding space where nerves are running. It may cause irritation of the nerve to a leg. This is called sciatica. The second most common disc to degenerate is the L4-5 disc. The upper lumbar discs are less common sites for degeneration than the lower ones. The lower lumbar spine not only degenerates more frequently than other parts of the lumbar spine, but it also experiences enormous physical stress on a day-to-day basis. Increased stress in the low lumbar spine happens to us all: there is no escape!

Low lumbar stresses occur in the soft tissues which surround bones and disc. These are mainly the ligaments and tendons which connect to the muscles that move the spine. Chronic strain or stress on these pain-sensitive structures is the usual cause for intermittent low back pain.

Just behind the lumbar vertebrae is the spinal canal — a gap between the vertebrae and the front of the bones forming the joints at the back — which allows the spinal nerves to run down to the lower parts of the body and the legs. Behind the spinal canal are the bony structures which make the back wall of the spinal canal and which connect to form the joints. The joints allow the lumbar spine to move smoothly and guidedly. These joints are called facet joints, approximately equal to the size of the joints in our fingers. Facet joints are very important in back problems.

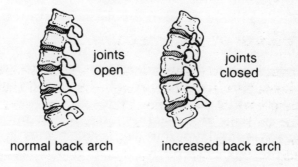

normal back arch   increased back arch

Figure 2 *Increased lowback arch gives tight joints*

The diagram (Figure 2) shows you that increased lordosis or arching of the lumbar spine will result in the facet joints 'closing down' and narrowing considerably. This puts enormous pressure on the outer lining of the joint, the capsule, perhaps causing stimulation of pain nerves in the joint capsule. Facet joints are positioned near the end of their normal range of motion (Figure 3).

Joint Action

Most joints in the body, such as the knuckle joint, allow

the two bones to sit in a neutral position, with plenty of movement downwards and upwards for the joint. This allows for plenty of play in the joint. In the facet joints of the low back, movement in one direction is minimal, but in another is much greater. The joint normally sits close to the end of its range of movement. This is the backward movement end. If further bending backwards occurs, the joint reaches the end of its normal range of motion. At this point, increased tissue pressure starts to act on the structures around the joint. This situation can be seen, for example, in the knuckle joint of the hand. Move the index finger as far as it will go, taking the joint to the end of its range. If you keep pushing the joint back and forth against that end range of motion, it will soon become painful (Figure 4). This is akin to what happens in the low back when the facet joint is at the end of its normal range of motion. The repetitive forces of everyday life, or the sudden jolts of a fall or a twist, will strain the joint and result in pain.

Situations that put the joint in this abnormally stressed position include postural hyperlordosis and degeneration of the discs of the low back. Degeneration of the discs will force pressure back on the joint. Hyperlordosis may occur through sports like gymnastics or serving in tennis. Hyperlordosis is sometimes a postural change present since birth. It may also relate to weak abdominal muscles or obesity. 'Pot belly' is the classic example of obesity. Here the centre of gravity moves forward. To maintain an upright position, the owner of this pot belly has to arch the back even further (Figure 5). This puts extra pressure on the facet joints and their sensitive linings, risking stimulation of the pain nerves. This is exactly what happens during pregnancy. As the baby grows up and out of the pelvis, a large pot belly occurs. The back arches and low back pain is common, especially later in the pregnancy.

Referred Pain

Once pain is generated from the pain-sensitive surround-

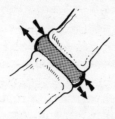

normal joint in mid part
of its ranged movement:
flexible

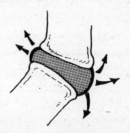

normal joint at extreme of
normal range: little movement
with marked increase in tension
on joint structures

Figure 3 *Normal joint: mid and extreme range*

ing structures of facet joints, then the pain is referred.
The other usual reflexes are also activated. You will
recall that any deep structure causing pain refers that
pain to the surface of the body, often some way from the
original pain site. Facet-joint pain from the low lumbar

---

*Jim was 52 and overweight. His low back
started to ache six months ago and was not
getting better. In the past he had had occasional
backaches, but they had never lasted this long.
The pain was in the middle of his low back and
radiated into his buttocks. It was worse towards
the end of the day, but improved a bit with rest.*

*Jim sought help. He found it in the form of
an exercise program (which also encouraged him
to lose some weight) and a short course of
anti-inflammatory medication. He has kept up
his level of exercise and kept down his weight.
Above all, he has accepted some responsibility for
his own health, his own needs.*

*Comment: Jim had developed mild
osteoarthritis of the small deep facet joints in the
low back. He was wise to choose exercise and*

*weight loss as the mainstays of his program.
Most episodes like Jim's, even though they
relate to an arthritis in the first instance, can be
handled well this way. 'Life — I'm now in it',
says Jim with some satisfaction!*

---

area usually brings pain across the low back or into the
upper buttocks, and sometimes down the back of the
legs. At times pain will even radiate into the lower leg and
towards the heel. Pain like this is usually a dull ache
rather than sharp and severe. This is classic rheumatism
of the low back, once termed lumbago.

Referred pain and other associated reflexes may be
made worse by stress, disturbed sleep, or other emotional

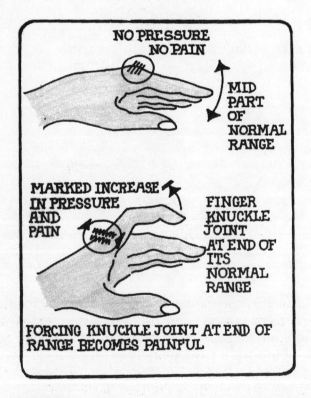

Figure 4

or psychological events. Greater local pain can occur, focusing on the low back. You are already aware that strain of the facet joints and other supporting ligaments and tendons can result in pain. This is not to say that they are actually damaged. With the young pregnant mother, her back ached quite a lot, but the joint was still very normal. It was just that the joint was in a bad or abnormal position. In other situations, more related to ageing than anything else, the facet joints may actually start to degenerate and become osteoarthritic (Figure 6).

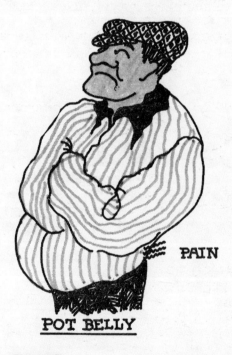

PAIN

POT BELLY

Figure 5

This is usually secondary to degeneration of the discs of the low back. As we age, osteoarthritic change in the lumbar spine is more common and more likely to be a source of low back pain, usually of an episodic nature. It is reassuring to know, however, that whilst most of us show x-ray degenerative changes in the low back, few of us have significant or long-term pain due to this.

Pain is also caused sometimes by other structures in the low back. Here we refer more specifically to damage or degeneration in the disc. This book does not aim to cover all these problems here. Briefly, though, the disc moves from its enclosed capsule and presses on nerves running in the spinal canal just behind the disc. Pressure of disc on nerve causes irritation of the nerve, with a resultant sharp and severe pain radiating down the nerve into the leg. This 'sciatic' pain is due to nerve root irritation. It's different to referred pain from facet joints and other structures in the low back, but sometimes the pain is inconclusive and needs special investigation to clarify the source of the pain.

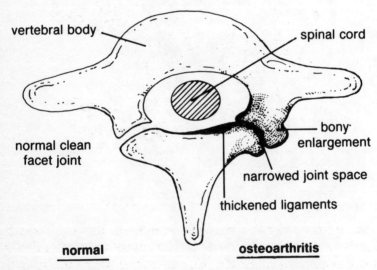

Figure 6 *Facet joint of the low back in health (L) and in sickness (R)*

Tests might include a computed x-ray tomography scan of the back to show the structure of the disc and its relationship to the large nerves and to the facet joint. Another test can be a myelogram: a needle is inserted into the space around the nerves, and dye is added to outline nerves and discs. Any disc that bulges out of place, with resultant pressuring of a nerve, will be seen.

Of all the causes of low back pain, most are caused by

strains and stresses around the facet joints. Only a few
can be blamed on disc disease and nerve root irritation.
Here, we are concerned with rheumatism rather than the
specific problems of nerve root irritation or disc disease.

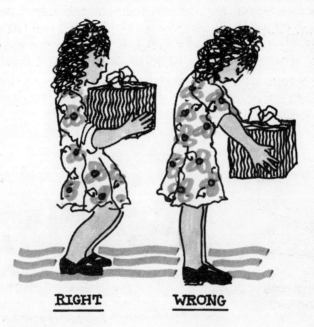

RIGHT   WRONG

Figure 7

Now let's refresh what has been said. Firstly, you are
now aware of the structure of the lumbar spine and why
spontaneous pain arises from postural abnormalities in
the lumbar spine. Spontaneous pain may be very local or
part of a more general fibrositis (which we shall discuss
later). Secondly, you may see low back pain as due to
degeneration of the disc or facet joint or to an injury to
one of these structures following trauma. All of these
problems may cause chronic intermittent back pain.

Then the focus was on acute and severe back pain —
usually due to strain on a supporting ligament, tendon or
joint lining; or to a small tear in the muscle from sudden
postural strain. Muscle tightness and even spasm can

occur. This protective muscle mechanism may cause its own degree of pain while the acute pain episode is going on.

What You Can Do

What do you do about low back pain? You must first start with an accurate diagnosis. This will entail a history and examination, and maybe some x-rays of the back. The extent of investigation by your doctor often relates to

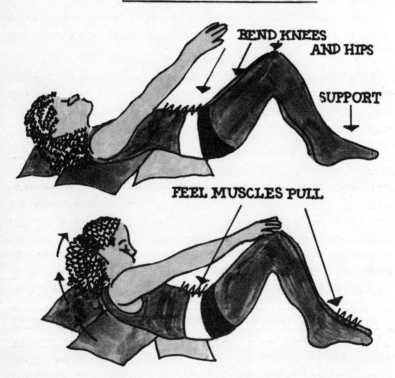

Figure 8

your age. For an elderly person with back pain, there are more possible causes. Let's suppose it's low back pain caused by postural effects on the facet joints and supporting structures, and there's resultant strain and stimulation of the pain nerves. The following treatments should then be considered.

• Back care is important. If the back aches, you should protect it. The do's and don'ts of low back care are well known to most sufferers. In essence, avoid bending or twisting with the back; instead bend with the knees and legs (Figure 7) and walk around objects rather than twist the spine. Train yourself not to do sudden movements with the back, but think before you move. As some people say, *Think back!* Carry heavy objects close to the body, and recognise that there is a limit to what you can do physically if your back is an ongoing problem. You usually know your limits, but sometimes you need to be told. It is hard to stop enjoyable activities, even if the back hurts!

• If you are over your ideal body weight, lose weight. Extra weight puts more strain on the structures of the back that are causing the pain. This goes without saying.

• Coupled with weight loss is strengthening your abdominal muscles. Firm abdominal muscles are important. Not only does this keep the centre of gravity towards the spine and not away from it, but it increases the strength of the muscles and the pressure within the abdominal cavity. This pressure acts in turn on the lumbar spine, preventing hyperlordosis and facet joint strain that can often occur near the end of a long day when muscles tire. Exercises to strengthen tummy muscles should be done with knees and hips bent and feet supported by a piece of furniture or a partner (Figure 8). This avoids excessive strain on the back — the thing you are trying to avoid like the plague! To begin these exercises, do the half sit-up rather than the full. Five to ten of these are enough for the first few days. Other ways to avoid hyperlordosis and strain on the back include standing with one foot slightly elevated — just like a drinker at the bar! This helps straighten the low back and eases pressure on pain-sensitive structures. Change position often during the day, and avoid holding the same posture for long periods.

● There are other exercises to strengthen muscles around the spine. These are usually best given by a physical therapist or exercise specialist. One exercise may be rotational: hips and knees bent up, knees on the tummy, you lying on your back. Rotate your knees from side to side (Figure 9). This stretches the tight areas in the low back which occur when pain is coming from the facet joint. It also stretches muscles, ligaments and joints, loosening up painful tight segments in the low back. Remember that with deep pain comes muscle tightness. This must be corrected.

Exercise Can Be a Winner

Regular exercise can help this program. Swimming is very good. It's a physical activity that does not put weight on the back, and the stretching and rotational movements of swimming help to loosen up the low back. Avoid

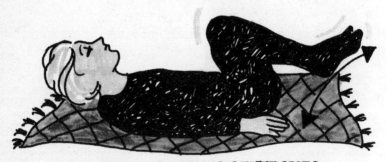

LOW BACK ROTATION EXERCISES

Figure 9

swimming strokes — like the butterfly and breaststroke — which tend to arch the back. Side stroke or back stroke are better, or do a gentle freestyle. So be wary of any exercise program that emphasises increased extension or bowing of the low back. The pelvic tilt works well. For this you lie on your back, knees bent, and try to make the back of your spine touch the floor by tilting the pelvis

PELVIC TILT EXERCISES

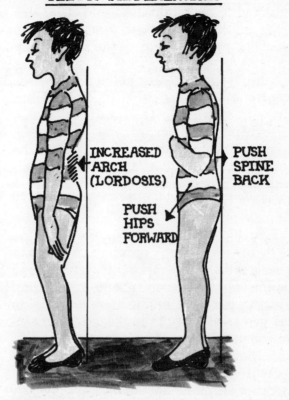

INCREASED
ARCH
(LORDOSIS)

PUSH
SPINE
BACK

PUSH
HIPS
FORWARD

Figure 10

back and forth — or do it standing up (Figure 10).

Don't forget the good advice that your bed should give you firm support, but not be rock-hard. Above all it must be comfortable. In general a standard, well made and firm mattress will be suitable to most.

If you see your doctor about back pain, you may be advised to take anti-inflammatory medication. It is used when there is inflammation in joints or soft tissues, and when you want pain relief that lasts twelve hours or so. Such medication is simple, safe and usually effective. But it won't cure postural back pain, just relieve the symptoms for a while.

Other treatments may be needed for a situation that lasts. Pain and tissue tenderness, and other signs of local or general fibrositis, require a different approach to management. This includes many of the suggestions made in Chapter 9.

All this discussion has been about posture-related, and usually chronic, low back pain. Sudden low back pain is usually due to a strain or tear in one of the supporting structures deep in the back. Maybe a disc prolapse is the culprit. In any event, the best treatment for it is rest. Rest means rest — not just saying you are going to rest! Go to bed. The problem will resolve itself in hours, days or even weeks! Let's say that if unfamiliar low back pain does not ease after a few days, talk to your doctor.

The low back is beautifully simple in its design and complex in its detail. Many different problems can affect the low back, most due to mechanical changes at the back of the spine. Degeneration in one area often leads to change in another area, and it may be the second structure that gives the symptoms. Conditions such as disc prolapse or herniation, disc degeneration, facet joint arthritis, spondylosis, spondylolisthesis, osteophytic impingement, ligamentous hypertrophy, spinal canal stenosis, scoliosis and a host of others may occur. These are usually problems of the older back.

By far the commonest back complaints relate to those discussed in this chapter. Attending to them is very important: they may need very different approaches to the basic back rules. They certainly need skilled assessment — by your doctor, sometimes by specialists, and by other health professionals. An individual program for each problem is needed. Nevertheless anyone with back pain can benefit from understanding the simple do's and don'ts of back care.

5

Fibrositis

The term *fibrositis* has been around for a long time. It was first coined in 1904 by an English doctor — Dr Gower. He was trying to understand the causes of low back pain or lumbago. Many patients with low back pain, he noted, had not only tenderness in the tissues but also thickening and nodules in the fatty layers under the skin. Dr Gower felt this was inflammation in the fibrous tissues — hence his new word 'fibrositis'. Unfortunately his observation and deductions were wrong. Other studies under the microscope of these fatty and painful nodules in the low back did not agree with Dr Gower's.

The term 'fibrositis' fell into medical disfavour. In fact for many years some health professionals have used the word to describe any ache or pain they can't easily explain. Others abandoned the term altogether, using different names to describe pain in the soft tissues.

So, despite years of controversy, the word 'fibrositis' continues in use, and over time many important observations have been brought together. These observations reached a climax in the mid 1970s when Professor Hugh Smythe from Toronto described the things that made up fibrositis, also known as fibrositis syndrome.

Research Has Big Benefits

Since then, lots of research has been carried out. Fibrositis has been classified and related to other rheumatic disorders. We now have a series of steps to follow in diagnosing it, thus separating fibrositis from other rheumatic conditions. And, most important of all, there has been a dramatic increase in research into the causes of fibrositis. However, in spite of all this progress, fibrositis still remains a mystery. Even though we know it is a predictable parcel of symptoms and signs, the actual cause remains hidden.

Yet fibrositis is the most common cause of chronic rheumatic complaints. It is present in all ages. It is the basic condition around which most rheumatic complaints revolve. Understanding fibrositis is the key to most rheumatic complaints.

Any word with 'itis' tagged on to the end means that inflammation is a large part of the cause. Words like arthritis, tonsillitis and appendicitis tell us that inflammation in those tissues causes the problem. However, we lack proof that inflammation, in the traditional sense, is part of fibrositis. So doctors have added the word syndrome to the title, making up the term 'fibrositis syndrome', but let's stick with fibrositis. It's simpler.

Some writers say other names should be used, e.g. muscle tension rheumatism, fibromyalgia, myofascial pain, and others. The most common alternative name now is fibromyalgia ('aching tissues'). Fibromyalgia, they argue, describes the main feature — a painful aching in the tissues — without hinting at any cause for the problem.

Now, fibrositis tends to affect more females than males, particularly through the late teens, the 20s, the 30s and into the 40s. Children can get the condition, but the adolescent years are more likely. It's less common for middle aged and older age groups to get fibrositis suddenly. Rather, they may have had a mild problem for many years — ready for it to worsen in later life!

Symptoms of Fibrositis

● Pain is the main complaint. Pain can vary quite a bit. It is usually felt in the spine, especially in the lower part of the neck and between the shoulder blades, the low back and buttocks, and also around the chest wall. The elbow, forearm, hand, knee and ankle are other places. The pain may be severe, but more likely a dull aching or burning.

● Muscle stiffness is the second characteristic — occurring at times around the spine, neck and low back. Some people get really stiff across the shoulders, down into the arms and all around the chest wall. The stiffness can come and go. Some people mainly have stiffness; others mainly pain; yet others have both. Stiffness is at its worst in the morning, perhaps eased by exercise, movement and heat.

● The other big problem is tiredness. This varies through the day, through the week or over many months. At times fatigue is the worst feature; at other times it's only a minor nuisance.

Pain, stiffness and fatigue vary a lot in different people. Each fluctuates quite markedly. At times there may be no symptoms, then for no obvious reason great tiredness or pain or stiffness occurs. This can last for some days or weeks, then start to wane. These episodes may persist over many weeks, months or even years.

Symptoms tend to start gradually, not abruptly — affected by factors like weather, physical activity, pos-

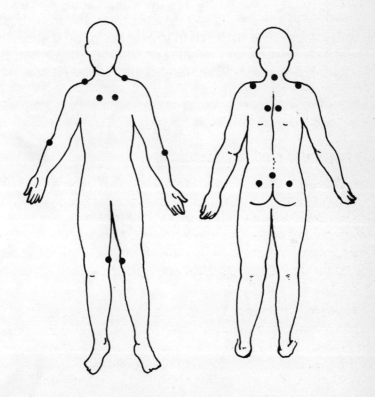

Figure 1 *Common tender points in fibrositis*

ture and emotional stress. Muggy or humid days, or weather associated with changes in barometric pressure, often precipitate symptoms. Stable dry, even if cold, air may be all right. Vigorous activity can stir up symptoms, either generally or in one part of the body. Don't be surprised if a big burst of house cleaning leads to stiffening and aching around the shoulders. Emotional stress is very crucial, yet difficult to quantify or identify in the comings and goings of everyday life. It's more common to find chronic low-grade stress (or unresolved conflict!) than sudden or severe stress. Worry about house payments may be more important than a severe accident for some people. As we said earlier, stresses vary as much as people.

Other signs of fibrositis are fluid retention, puffiness or swelling of the hands — particularly in the mornings. Rings tighten. The strength of grip in the hand is weaker. There may be pins and needles or tingling in the hands, particularly at night. The hand feels numb. Headaches

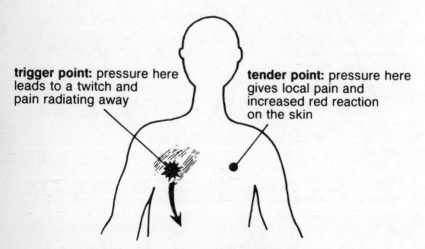

trigger point: pressure here leads to a twitch and pain radiating away

tender point: pressure here gives local pain and increased red reaction on the skin

Figure 2 *Trigger points versus tender points*

commonly occur: 'tension headaches' or more like a migraine. They are usually at the back of the neck or over the top of the head, maybe lasting for days or weeks.

Other people have an irritable bowel with constipation or diarrhoea and irregular bowel habit, abdominal bloating and discomfort.

When fibrositis is diagnosed, the doctor must make sure it is not an underlying condition mimicking fibrositis. For example, people with low thyroid hormone levels commonly have muscle aches. Thyroid hormone helps to maintain the energy balance of the body, and it may be wise to test for abnormalities in thyroid hormones when assessing muscular pain and fatigue. Many other systemic illnesses — e.g. infections, mineral metabolism abnormalities, or more serious conditions like cancer — can produce general muscular aching and pain. A list of problems which mimic the symptoms of fibrositis is shown in the table.

Referred pain is also tricky. Remember that it can cause stiffness, aching and pain in the arm and muscles, and mimic the symptoms of fibrositis.

Signs of Fibrositis

The first checks are to see there are no abnormalities in the body's systems — heart, lungs, kidneys, gastrointestinal and hormone systems — and no changes in any of the organs. The joints must move normally, even if sometimes stiffly and with pain. There should be no sign of inflammation in joints (showing up as swelling or redness over the joints), nor any abnormality on testing the major nerves or the muscles.

● *Tender points* are important. Figure 1 shows the common tender points seen in fibrositis. The diagram is really a summary of the many tender points observed in fibrositis. They are the ones most useful in diagnosis. A tender point is an area in the soft tissues or along bony prominences. When pressed, there is more pain than from similar pressure to a nearby spot. This is a long-winded way of saying that tender points hurt more than other points.

Tender points are similar, but not identical, to trigger points. Trigger points occur in muscles under certain cir-

MIMICS OF FIBROSITIS

1. MECHANICAL PROBLEM IN SPINE. (LEADING TO REFERRED PAIN)

2. INFLAMMATORY ARTHRITIS.

3. WIDESPREAD DEGENERATIVE ARTHRITIS.

4. POLYMYALGIA RHEUMATICA.

5. HORMONAL DISORDER E.G. THYROID LOW.

6. MALIGNANCY.

7. OTHER.

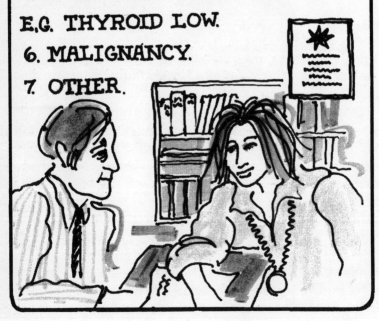

cumstances. Pressure to a trigger point causes pain, and it radiates in a way which exactly imitates the complaint. Trigger points occur in a single muscle, but fibrositis may involve many muscles (Figure 2). You all have tender points, even when you do not have symptoms of generalised aching. Try the pinch test. Grip the middle of the main muscle between the neck and shoulder, and give it a slight pinch. It's more sensitive than adjacent areas even

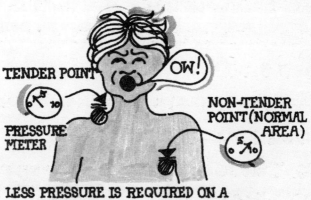

Figure 3

a few centimetres away from the pinch or tender point. You are also tender just below the bony point of the elbow, in the upper forearm. This is more prone to tenderness than nearby parts. Indeed all the typical tender points in Figure 1 are spots where less stimulation is needed to cause discomfort or pain. In people with fibrositis, the tenderness at these points is more marked than is usual in those without symptoms. In Canada they have shown this very clearly by use of pain-pressure meters. Look at Figure 3 and you will see this vividly in a diagram.

Tender points cause confusion and controversy among doctors. Many argue that the signs are not valid because you can't see anything! However, when you consider all the different signs, you appreciate that tenderness is a very important clinical sign. Which doctor would diagnose appendicitis and operate on a patient who was not tender over the appendix area?

● The second major finding in people with fibrositis is *dermatographia* or red-flare reaction. This means that the skin reacts more to gentle stimulation than it would otherwise do. For example, if the skin between the shoulder blades is scratched with a fingernail, a red line appears after a short while. The line traces the path the nail took. This is normal. In patients with fibrositis, the same scratch results in greater red reaction, even producing some slight swelling where the nail has passed over the skin. This is called dermatographia (Figure 4).

● Varied reactions are seen in people without fibrositis. Some react a lot, others very little. But patients with fibrositis react much more. Overlap does exist between some normal people and some people with fibrositis. This is also true of the tender points. Some patients without signs have tender points as sensitive as those in people with fibrositis. These are the exception. Yet it

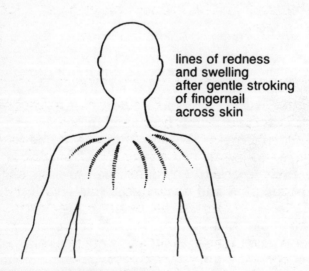

lines of redness
and swelling
after gentle stroking
of fingernail
across skin

Figure 4 *Dermatographia*

does tell us that these physical findings are linked with fibrositis, though they are not necessarily the cause. As you will see later, they are a major clue to understanding the condition.

● People with fibrositis also get *muscle stiffness*, especially around the neck and shoulder. When these muscles move normally, it's usual for different muscle groups to contract and relax in a rhythmic way. In people with fibrositis, muscles often tighten in odd ways and are difficult to relax — say, when the arm moves in the opposite direction.

These then are the features of fibrositis. It is so important to establish that there is no underlying condition which can copy the symptoms of fibrositis. However, fibrositis is very common and usually it's possible to confirm its presence quickly. The typical complaints described here are those of so-called *primary fibrositis*. Primary means there is no other underlying cause. In other words, there has been no injury or dramatic event that preceded the symptoms. The signs have merely shown up over time and for no apparent reason. Sometimes fibrositis occurs with or after an identifiable event — for instance, a car accident or a work injury or a death in the family. This is called *secondary fibrositis*, and it is discussed later.

A twenty-nine-year old, Kirsten was a teacher at a technical college. Early in the year she developed a severe flu-like illness that lasted for several weeks. She had a cough, general malaise, low grade fever and a rash for a time. Later she developed joint and muscle pain, general muscle weakness and fatigue. She began to sleep very poorly.

Until then Kirsten had been very well. She led an active life — she played tennis, went hiking and swam, regularly. She had been doing a PhD for some years and, all in all, had a hectic schedule.

Her flu-like symptoms disappeared, but she was left with fatigue, general muscle weakness and aching, and a feeling of stiffness, particularly in the morning. Her hands often felt numb or tingly during the night; her sleep was unrefreshing and then her head felt foggy through the day. She was having trouble concentrating and continuing her part-time study. Physical activity, such as playing tennis, aggravated her symptoms, so she stopped them.

Because of these complaints, it was decided that Kirsten should have some tests. The hunt was on for a persistent undefined virus or other general illness, so she saw lots of doctors and other health professionals. But her symptoms lasted despite various medications and treatments.

Kirsten had developed fibrositis.

There was no abnormality on general examination, but she did have tender points in the usual areas, as well as muscle stiffness in the neck, low back and shoulders. She had dermatographia when the skin on her back was lightly stroked, and even when the skin over the upper back was pinched she would have pain.

Her problem was explained to Kirsten, as well as the importance of exercise and relaxation. She was given a low dose of an antidepressant medication for sleep disturbance, started regular exercise again, and reviewed her commitments in life. She took up relaxation techniques. Her problem fluctuated for some time — with good days and bad days, often precipitated by weather change.

Some two years after the initial diagnosis, Kirsten wrote:

Physically, life is often a bit of a battle for me. I still get lots of joint pain, although nowadays I can control the soft tissue hurt by conscious efforts, but the pain in the bones can be really hard to live with. I get very tired too — although everyone assures me I still achieve more than average (whatever that means!). However, after first having a fairly traumatic period, I seem to have come to terms with it all. I've got back most of my old enthusiasm for life and, much to my relief, my brain seems to work again (a completely subjective opinion)! It's great to be back home making new friends, enjoying the climate — until this summer heat which is awful — and being fully committed to my job. Let me reassure you, though, that I participate in everything with a little reserve. I have learnt to keep a little energy for myself. I continue to meditate, walk in the countryside near home every day, and swim several times a week. All in all, life's okay!

Comment: Kirsten's situation is fairly typical of a severe episode of fibrositis. Note that she was quite well before this came on. It was triggered by an apparent viral illness, but it started in the midst of big life commitments in someone who was highly motivated and of the high achieving type. It was a piece of straw that broke the camel's back. The pain pathways became activated and fibrositis resulted.

Her progress was slow but steady. She improved a lot but still suffered significant symptoms from time to time. The main message here is that she has come to terms with her problem and is learning to live with it. She has not lost all her symptoms but with more time further improvement will occur. As Kirsten said, 'All in all life's okay!'

Understanding Fibrositis

You can make close comparisons between the symptoms
and signs of fibrositis and those of deep referred pain
from spinal structures. It is also true that most symptoms in people with fibrositis occur in the lower neck and
back and in areas which relate to those regions — such as
the shoulder, chest, upper back, buttocks and legs. You
will also see (from Figure 5) that the tender points cluster
around the neck and low back.

The lowest vertebral segments of the neck (the cervical spine) and the back (the lumbar spine) are the
places where most wear and tear occur. This has much to
do with our upright posture, and the shape of the bones,
discs and supporting structures in those regions. For
simple mechanical reasons, these areas have to with-
stand big physical stresses. As we discussed, joints and
other tissues function in a compromised way — at the
limits of mechanical resistance. With time, degenerative
changes occur in the discs and later in the joints of these
parts of the spine. But even at younger ages, when there
are no signs on x-rays or elsewhere, stresses still occur in
the lower neck and back during everyday activities.

Look again at the types of pain caused by defects in
deep spinal structures. This way you can build up a picture of fibrositis. Deep pain in the low neck is referred
down the arm, leading to various kinds of pain. It can also
cause a sensation of tingling in the hand, numbness and
swelling. Also, as you saw earlier, the same single source
of pain leads to referred tenderness in predictable spots
quite distant from the initial problem. Tenderness is
common in the middle of the trapezius muscle, the inner
shoulder blade, the front of the chest wall, in the
shoulder itself, the outer elbow, and the main web
between thumb and first finger (Figure 6). Muscles
tighten and become stiff. The same central source of
deep pain causes reflex changes — through the nervous
system — to the flow of blood to the skin of the upper
back and to the arm. In some people an unusual 'chicken-
wire' rash appears on the front of the forearm, or the

palm becomes red.

Over the upper back marked dermatographia is seen. The same occurs with deep pain from the low back. Here, as in the neck, symptoms and signs are identical to those seen in fibrositis, except that they occur in the back, buttocks and legs.

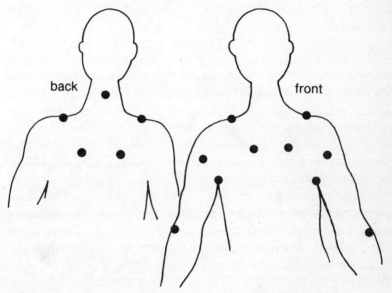

Figure 5 *Clustering of tender points around the neck*

Pain Amplification

So the symptoms and signs of fibrositis can be explained by reflex pain from deep pain low in the neck and back — areas already under great mechanical stress in the normal person. The current idea is that fibrositis is caused mainly by a *pain amplification*. This means that pain pathways and nerve reflexes are amplified and become very sensitive. These amplified pathways are normal pain nerve pathways that are activated by simple mechanical stresses present in all of our spines.

Recent evidence suggests that there is indeed activation of normal pain pathways and reflexes in people with fibrositis. If you apply the chemical Capsaicin to the skin (it's a close relative of the Hungarian red pepper), this chemical activates and stimulates the pain nerve fibres. It does not affect any other nerve fibres in the skin. Activating the pain nerve fibres releases the chemical substance P, making more blood flow into the skin.

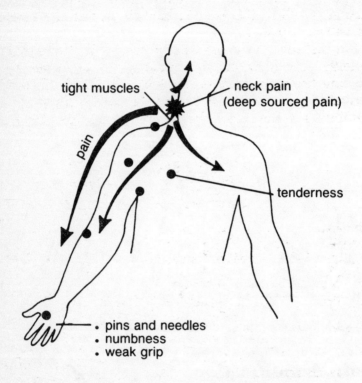

Figure 6 *Strain deep in neck giving rise to automatic reflex 'referred' pain*

This causes the red reaction of the skin — equivalent to the dermatographia reaction seen when the skin is stroked with a fingernail. Researchers have studied this reaction and found that, in people with fibrositis, the small pain nerve fibres in the skin react much more than in normal people without aches and pains and without tender points (i.e. without fibrositis). There is a close relationship between this reaction and the number of tender points in someone with fibrositis. The more tender points there are, the more red reaction of the skin. This suggests that these two events are linked through the nervous system.

This idea is most exciting. For the first time it shows that the pain-nerve system is stirred up and amplified in people with fibrositis. It is likely then that many other changes in fibrositis are also due to activation of reflex nerve reactions.

For instance, if the pain-nerve system is stimulated, it reflexly acts back on the muscles in the same area, causing them to tighten and feel stiff. With fibrositis, activated pain nerves may also cause the tingling and numbness in the hands. Remember that, when the skin

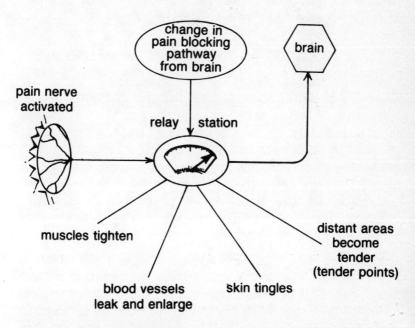

Figure 7 *Reflex activation of many nerves occurs in fibrositis*

touch sensation is tested in fibrositis, it is normal; but of course sensation goes along different pathways to the pain nerves themselves. So the abnormal sensations seem to relate to the pain nerves alone. Further activation of the pain system may also cause reflex reactions on blood vessels and make them react abnormally; this can cause them to expand, leak fluid and give the sensation of tissue swelling. All this helps to explain the tightening of rings in such people. The diagram (Figure 7) illustrates how these reactions occur.

The muscles of people with fibrositis look normal under the microscope. However, when examined by a very powerful electron microscope, very subtle changes can be seen. These changes are not special to fibrositis: they can happen with other painful muscle conditions. More recent studies reveal changes in the metabolism of fibrositic muscles. Such muscles use oxygen and other nutrients in a different way. Maybe these changes are also reflex reactions on the muscles, and occur as automatic reactions to stimulating pain nerves.

Two Key Factors

There is a strong case for explaining fibrositis as the activation of reflex nerve-fibre pathways. These reflexes seem to focus in the low neck and low back, where things are already under stress and strain. How then is the pain made worse? Psychological factors are important. Emotional tension and other psychological factors lead to activation of the pain nerve pathways, this writer believes. The abnormality caused results in the symptoms and signs of fibrositis.

● People with fibrositis sleep poorly. Their sleep is shallow. They toss and turn through the night, and wake unrefreshed. It is common for sleep disturbance to precede the problem. With the return of even sleep, muscle symptoms often settle. Doctors Moldofsky and Smythe tested this in the 1970s. They found that, by measuring the brain waves of people with fibrositis, they could identify a typical pattern. Normally during sleep the brainwaves slow down and show a 'delta' pattern. Those with fibrositis had a 'delta' pattern all right, but as well they had a rapid 'alpha' waking pattern which intruded

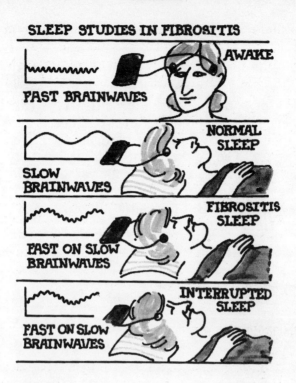

Figure 8

into the normal slow wave delta sleep. This is the so-called 'alpha-delta' sleep pattern (Figure 8). Again it is not exclusive to fibrositis, but it seems characteristic.

The two researchers then studied normal medical students without aches or pains. They measured the students' brainwave patterns in the sleep laboratory — disrupting their sleep regularly without wakening them — for several nights. Doing this, they mimicked the 'alpha-delta' sleep brainwave pattern seen in fibrositis patients. The 'normal' medical students began to ache and develop tenderness in the predictable tender point areas seen in fibrositis. They became tired and, in effect, developed fibrositis. Sleep abnormality, it was decided, was important. It probably happened before the fibrositis, rather than being just a problem for someone with lots of aches and pains and who can't sleep well. This is the first clue that psychological factors are important in fibrositis.

● The second major clue is the link between fibrositis and life's stresses. It is usual to find a very stressful event in the life of someone with fibrositis. This can be an obvious event (say, the death of a partner), or perhaps something more subtle and even longer lasting (e.g. conflict at work). People with fibrositis are usually high-achieving, meticulous and well motivated people. They tend to be more anxious and concerned, although this is not always the case. But fibrositis sufferers are not more depressed than others.

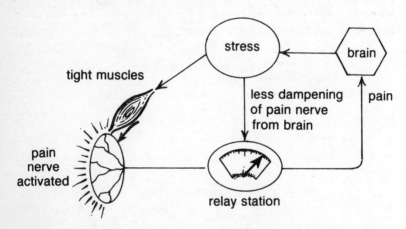

Figure 9 *Effects of stress on pain system*

Numerous scientific studies have been done to try to work out the typical profile of a person with fibrositis. However, as yet the picture is not clear. But you can say that people with fibrositis are more prone to other stress-linked problems — such as irritable bowel, tension headache and menstrual irregularities. Sometimes fibrositis is suspected by the bad company it keeps!

So we have mechanical pain pathway factors and psychological stress factors. One way to bring these two things together is to recall the basic pain pathways. Any pain message which reaches the spinal cord of the nervous system is influenced by other nerve impulses from the brain and also the muscles. These impulses influence the incoming 'pain' at the relay station. The pain sensation is modified before it proceeds further into the nervous system (i.e. up to the brain) and thus to the level of consciousness or feeling (Figure 9).

Psychological and stress factors probably change the normal control of pain, exaggerating it and enabling reflex phenomena to start. Once the regular system has changed, it takes a lot of retraining for the normal dampening and inhibition of the system to be fixed.

Very often the *original* stress or trigger which changed the system may have resolved itself, but the symptoms persist. This is because of a change in 'setting' the central nervous system as it deals with the pain. The 'setting' needs to be turned down by other means.

6

Localised Fibrositis

You heard about the features of fibrositis in the last chapter. Let's focus now on localised forms of fibrositis and other variations on the same fibrositis theme.

Work and Fibrositis

Jenny was forty-eight when she first complained about generalised musculoskeletal pain. She had pain in the low back, the buttocks, the right hip, the inner side of the knees, the low neck, the upper back, the shoulders and around the elbow. Her pain came and went — severe at times, at other times not so bad. Sometimes she had trouble taking deep breaths due to chest wall pain. At other times she would have trouble on the toilet because of right buttock pain. She had numbness in the arms and hands at night. The pain was worse with weather changes, particularly humid weather. Physical activity made the pain worse too. Jenny often had a sensation of swelling in her hands although no one could see any swelling.

Jenny had had many years of irregular periods and irritable bowels, with bloating of her abdomen from time to time. She could not tolerate anti-inflammatory tablets: they tended to upset her stomach very easily.

She had fibrositis. She had the tender points in the usual areas, but everything else was normal.

The complication in Jenny's case was that she felt that work had caused her problem. She definitely felt worse through the day, particularly when she was sitting at her desk. At work the more she thought about it, the more she ached. Because of this, she put in a compensation claim for an injury induced at work. Since then she has had treatments by different therapists, taken

*numerous kinds of tablets and been seen by
several doctors. No one was able to tell her why
she was aching. She was reassured there was
nothing wrong, but she did not accept the
reassurance. She still ached so much and felt so
bad. In the end Jenny left work because of the
problem, yet in spite of being away from the
place she blamed for the problem, she got worse.*

*Comment: Jenny had fibrositis. It was not
caused by work. It was not caused by the shape
of the chair, the position of the desk, the air
conditioner set up in the office, or any other
physical feature of the place. It was the physical
condition at work she had been blaming. In fact,
after some discussion, it turned out that she had
a number of problems with her boss at work, and
there were large conflicts that she could not face.
She had always been a bit achy, but the office
environment brought things to a head.*

There are real dangers in blaming fibrositis symptoms
on work. It is common for people to go from doctor to
doctor seeking the magic cure. Doctors may either not
recognise fibrositis or they may attribute the symptoms
to other reasons, initiating lots of tests and treatments
which fail. In addition there will be a legal argument
about cause and effect. It's common for the sufferer of
fibrositis to go from the insurance company doctors to
the solicitor's doctors in order to gather reports and to be
put through the mill. All of this greatly aggravates the
fibrositis.

The answer is to get back to work, to stop compensation proceedings and to adopt correct management principles. Fibrositis is not an injury. It does not respond to
treatment as an injury. If it is so treated, fibrositis will set
in for a long time. The disruption to life will be major.
Yet, unfortunately, this is an all too common situation
nowadays.

Fibrositis and Arthritis

Kim was thirty-four when she found she had rheumatoid arthritis. She developed swelling and pain in the small joints of her hands and feet. She had difficulty in doing lots of everyday things, including looking after her two young children. She began anti-inflammatory medication and improved quite a bit. The disease fluctuated from time to time, but she could do most things without much discomfort.

One year later, she developed general aches and pains, fatigue and stiffening in the mornings. She was sleeping poorly. Her husband had lost his job, and there were money problems in the family. Her increased joint and muscle pain were blamed on arthritis, and she was changed from her tablets to others. These did not help her. She went through numerous treatments including injections — but to no avail. In fact she had developed fibrositis. When this was realised and clearly differentiated from the features of her arthritis, she responded to the right treatment and is now much better.

It's so common for patients with arthritis, or indeed any other chronic illness, to develop fibrositis. There is the danger too that the symptoms of the fibrositis will be similar to those of the arthritis. The conditions can be easily separated on clinical examination, but an unsuspecting observer may not recognise the important difference. If fibrositis is not properly diagnosed in someone who has an underlying arthritis, then the wrong treatment can be given for the symptoms. This of course is true for many conditions where the symptoms of fibrositis mimic those of an already existing illness. In fact fibrositis keeps company with a whole host of conditions, particularly arthritis.

On the other hand, some people with fibrositis are diagnosed as having an arthritis. This of course is quite wrong. They are then given wrong treatment and wrong advice.

Injury and Fibrositis

Clare was thirty-two. She entertained regularly, helped on the school council and had a part-time job. She was well liked by her friends and had a very good marriage. Always well dressed and well groomed, she liked to do her best at everything.

One day whilst driving her children home from school, she was stationary at the traffic lights when a van ran into the back of her car. She was jolted but did not hit anything. Next day she awakened with her neck aching; the ache continued over another day or so, and got severe. Her neck became stiff. The pain extended into the shoulders, down the back and around the chest wall. She was told it would go away within a few weeks.

Clare's problem lasted for months. She was told she had 'whiplash'. The pain got worse, there was muscle stiffness, her sleep became disturbed and her hands became numb at night. She tended to drop things very easily. She became nervous and lost confidence. She withdrew and lost friends, her marriage became strained and she lost control. She had tender points around the neck and chest and arm, but nowhere else in the body. She had developed localised fibrositis.

When the soft tissues of the neck are injured, as occurs

in common end-to-end collisions or other minor accidents, there is usually a neck ache for some days or even
for a few weeks. The soft tissues heal in a number of days
or weeks. Six to eight weeks is the maximal healing time.
The soft tissue pain that occurs within that first six
weeks is often popularly called 'whiplash'.

Pain which occurs in the same tissues after that is
usually due to the onset of fibrositis. The activated pain
pathways occur locally and cause localised fibrositis, and
they may lead to just so many investigations and treatments before the right diagnosis is made.

About 20 percent of minor motor car accidents lead to
this type of fibrositis, often after a very trivial injury.
Even though the physical injury is trivial, the psychological injury can be great. Traffic accidents are scary, and
they do play on the mind for a long time. It's very important to tackle the emotional and worry bits of such problems right from the start. Try to nip them in the bud!
This is much more sensible than a host of medications or
physical treatments of the soft tissues.

Adolescent Fibrositis

*Anna was fourteen when she developed pain in
joints and muscles. For many years she had had
headaches. She felt poorly and slept poorly. She
was usually exhausted at night and went to bed
early. Despite this she could not get a good
night's sleep. Examination showed her to have
fibrositis. She started an exercise program and
some of the stresses in her life were addressed.
These related to problems at school and some
interactive problems at home. A skilled clinical
psychologist saw her and offered good practical
advice. Six months later she was symptom-free
and coping well.*

Generalised fibrositis is common in adolescents, particularly females. It is usually of a minor or trivial type, but at times it does need consultation with a doctor. There is often unresolved stress in the background that requires proper management, then the outcome is usually very good. Fibrositis in children and adolescents is the same as that in adults.

Low Back Pain and Fibrositis

Jim was 28. He had worked for seven years on the factory floor. He was used to lifting heavy loads. One day he felt his back 'give'. He had muscle spasm and rested from work for ten days. His x-rays were normal. He had physiotherapy and medication, but did not get any better. His pain continued, and he stayed off work for several months. He had developed localised fibrositis in the low back. Further treatment for Jim consisted of an exercise program and careful explanation of the problem. He needed to be reassured that there was no ongoing tissue damage or injury, as he had suspected. Jim was given careful counselling by a work rehabilitationist, eventually returning to his full normal life.

Low back fibrositis is more common in men. Often localised, it follows something like a simple muscle or ligament tear that otherwise heals in its own time. Persistence of the pain usually reflects fear of a hidden deeper injury that has been missed by doctors or other people. There are lots of myths about backs in the community, and money compensation can loom large. Such problems are less common in the self-employed, who tend to put aside minor aches and get back to work as

soon as possible, not allowing the pain amplification
pathways to become activated. It's too bad that patients
with low back fibrositis are often prescribed long periods
of rest, rather than active exercise and a back re-
education program.

Arm Pain and Fibrositis

*Chris was a typist. She was happy with her
typewriter, but a new word processor was brought
in. Other women in the office began to complain
of pain in the wrist with the newer word
processors, and she worried that she might
develop the same problem. She did. However, the
pain in the wrist did not stay there. It spread
into the forearm and up into the neck. She could
not continue her job and had to leave work.
Despite this the pain got worse. Her hand felt
different and became numb and tingly. She
dropped things. Sometimes her hand swelled in
the mornings, even becoming a dusky colour. Her
neck was stiff. Generally fatigued through the
day, yet she slept poorly. She did not respond to
physiotherapy and reacted badly to different
tablets given to her.*

*Despite several months' rest the problem did
not go away. Chris had fibrositis. She was very
sensitive in the tender points of the neck, arm,
and between thumb and second finger. But in no
time at all she began to respond to explanation of
the problem, to reassurance about lack of tissue
damage or injury, and to a program of relaxation
and exercise. After some weeks she returned to
general office work, and then to her word
processor after some more months.*

*Comment: This is a particular type of localised
fibrositis known as regional pain syndrome.
During the working day there are many*

*opportunities for pain to occur in the arm or
neck. Poor posture, badly designed furniture or
office equipment itself may cause aching after a
certain amount of work. The risk is that pain
pathways will become activated, causing the
automatic reflex activity discussed earlier. A
simple ache can activate pathways that lead to
fibrositis. Worry, fear, tenseness and blaming
symptoms on others all add to pain amplification.
It is better to prevent this problem than treat it.
But to understand it is the best path to
treatment. Early return to work, exercise and
relaxation are the keys to treatment.*

There are many other examples of different types of
fibrositis, either general or local. A common thread runs
through all of them. One major danger of fibrositis is its
link sometimes with so-called secondary gain (e.g. work
compensation or sympathy). In these situations fibrositis can persist indefinitely while the problem remains
unresolved.

Epidemics of Fibrositis

Fibrositis is also prone to epidemics. After the wars there
has always been an epidemic of young men who come
home with generalised fibrositis, often called by such
other names as 'shell shock'. These young men have not
been physically damaged, but emotionally traumatised
by war. This has affected their pain pathways, giving rise
to fibrositis symptoms. Epidemics of fibrositis have also
occurred in some work places, usually affecting the low
back or arms. Such epidemics are fanned by bad publicity
through the media and by poor community understanding of the effects of stress, emotion and psychological
factors on physical symptoms. As a community, we must
be on guard against such epidemics.

With problems like fibrositis, where the cause is not apparent at the superficial level, there are always people prepared to give reasons for the problems. In the early 1950s, during the polio years, young nurses in hospitals often developed fibrositis. Again these outbreaks were often epidemics. None of the nurses developed polio, but their fibrositis persisted for years. This condition was called *myalgic encephalomyelitis*. It's a name devised to explain the symptoms the young women had, as if it was a probable viral infection. Of course this was never proved. It was also interesting that the symptoms cleared up completely with stress management and exercise. There will always be new names for different explanations of fibrositis — particularly when it occurs in epidemic proportions!

7

Tests and Rheumatism

Health professionals get most information about people by talking to them! This is sometimes forgotten. To diagnose a problem the health professional looks for a pattern of symptoms. The sequence of events, types of complaints, distribution of complaints, and the variation of symptoms — these all help as the pieces of the diagnostic puzzle are put together. The person's health history is so crucial in rheumatic disorders.

The next stage is examination of the person. It's often said that, with a good history and examination, most rheumatic complaints will be diagnosed. However, to help eliminate various possibilities, there is often a need for blood tests, x-rays, or other special tests. At times these tests will actually diagnose the disease or complaint.

Many common rheumatic complaints are so characteristic that talking to and examining the person will give the right answer. On the other hand, some rheumatic problems require a series of checks to make sure the diagnosis is spot on. Nowadays it is very easy for a doctor to perform a whole series of tests, taking up a lot of time, and be accused of ordering too many tests! It is vital to do *selective tests*, not general screening. Tests should be relevant to the ideas that come up in chatting about the complaints and examining the relevant areas. The more the tests in rheumatic diseases, the less the knowledge of the person ordering the tests!

X-ray Pictures

Complaints of pain or stiffness in the neck or back may mean an x-ray. X-rays say some important things. Take the neck. The bony outlines of the different bits of the neck show up very clearly. Often several x-rays are done at the one time — at different angles to show the joints, the back of the neck, and the disc spaces between the bones of the neck. As well, the exit holes for the nerves stand out on another routine x-ray view. So, by looking at a set of x-rays, you can get a picture of the anatomy of the neck.

● The only things that show on standard x-rays are bones (Figure 1). You do not see discs, cartilage of the joints, nerves, tendons, ligaments or muscles. You do not see soft tissues. In fact, you do not see that whole story — only changes that affect the bones. Disorders such as disc 'wear and tear' may lead to narrowing of the disc, and bones separated by the disc come closer together. You also see joints become narrow because cartilage lining the joint has worn down. You see bony spurs around joints, recognising this as a sign of osteoarthritis. So the first point to realise is that you are looking only at bony tissues — not visualising a whole host of 'soft tissues' which are the likely culprits in causing pain in the neck.

● The second thing about routine x-rays is that they confirm changes that occur naturally. For instance, as you progress through life, the discs in the lower neck start to narrow, and the spaces between the bones come closer to each other. The joints at the back of the spine — especially in the lowest part of the neck — also show signs of narrowing and of spurs, signs that point the finger at osteoarthritis. Thus it is common to see changes in the lower part of the neck in people as they age. These changes are noticeable from the mid-thirties on, sometimes earlier. It is on the cards that some people in their fifties will have changes on x-ray.

It is important to remember, though, that changes may sometimes *not* produce any symptoms at all. Indeed this is the usual situation — abnormal x-rays but no symptoms. When there's an x-ray of the neck of someone with pain or stiffness, you will probably find changes in the neck on x-ray. This is not to say that changes on x-ray are anything to do with the symptoms. Overinterpretation of x-rays leads to much unnecessary concern by patients and often overtreatment by health professionals. So the x-ray has to be taken into account with symptoms, examination findings and other factors.

The same comments apply to the low back. Wear and tear in the lowest part of the back — the lumbar spine — are also common and worsen with age. Another factor is

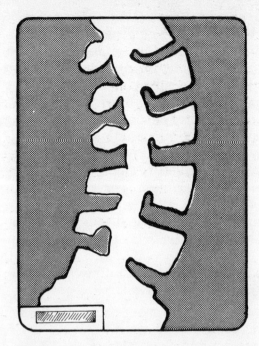

Figure 1 *X-ray of the spine*

important here. About 20 percent of people have abnormalities in the low back that are present from birth. These abnormalities persist through life, again usually without symptoms. They have such technical names as *spina bifida occulta* or sacralisation of the transverse process of the fifth lumbar vertebra. Overinterpretation of these findings must be avoided too.

In the mid-back, x-rays show up changes, known as Scheuermann's disease, in 20 percent of people after their teen years. Often present without symptoms, this may lead to x-ray changes seen later in life. These include narrowing of the disc and other changes around the disc. But they cannot be blamed as the cause of the pain that prompted the x-rays in the first place.

Another thing often seen on back x-rays are spurs of new bone forming at the front of the spinal column. *Idiopathic hyperostosis* is the name for this condition, and it's particularly common in heavy-set people or people who have mature-onset diabetes. Again the x-ray shows signs for which there are no symptoms.

Seen from the front, the spine in most people has a small irregularity in alignment. This is called *scoliosis*. At times it is severe and may also be painful, but for most people minor sideways curving of the spine does not matter. Once, chiropractors even measured the alignment of the spine and marked where adjustments were needed to cure the symptoms. Thankfully, this attitude has faded with time. Minor curvature changes in the spine are normal, and lengthy therapies to correct such deformities do not make for good health care.

So routine x-rays can yield lots of information, but interpret them carefully to avoid wrong meaning given to a normal finding. Only if x-ray findings tally with symptoms and examination findings should decisions be made on the basis of x-rays.

Newer Equipment and Tests

Different types of x-ray machines have been developed in recent years. The *computed tomography scan*, or CT scan, takes the radiological process a bit further. This device allows many soft tissue structures to be seen. The spine's soft tissues of interest include the disc, the spinal nerves, and some of the ligaments. The CT scan shows displacement of discs from their normal position — as well as abnormality of the main spinal nerves as they leave the lower back or neck — and distortions of other structures. The test is easy to perform, accurate but expensive. Approach the results with care: they may be normal for the patient's age and not contribute to symptoms. For instance, it's common to see discs bulging in the low back, yet not totally out of place. This is usually normal. As you learn more about normal changes with this sophisticated test, you will be better able to recognise abnormality. The CT scan is good at showing the structure of the small facet joints at the back of the spine, particularly in the low back. Remember that the facet joints are often the source of pain referred into buttocks or legs.

New scans — using even more sophisticated techniques — are also available. One of these, the magnetic resonance imaging or MRI machine, is very good at visualising the disc. Some interesting observations have been made in the United Kingdom using MRI. Significant disc deterioration was seen in twenty-year-old women. Between age twenty and forty, almost a third of women had abnormal discs in the low back. Yet none of the women in the study had symptoms. There were no complaints of back pain, even though the detailed picture was showing changes in the structure of the back. This further emphasises the big difference between structural changes of the body and actual symptoms. Change in structure usually does not cause symptoms. When the symptom is pain, this is very relevant.

There are other more invasive ways to assess spinal pain. A *myelogram* is such a test. A needle is inserted into the fluid space around the spinal nerves of the lower back. Dye is instilled, and x-rays are taken to show the outline of the spinal nerves. Needles can also be inserted into the disc space to show any deterioration. Because disc abnormalities are common, the investigator tries to reproduce the exact pain of which the patient complains.

In other areas, x-rays give similar images of the bone and of the space between the bones (i.e. the joint cartilage). X-rays can show joint space narrowing and bony spurs typical of osteoarthritis, or other arthritic changes affecting the joint space. Although many kinds of arthritis have very characteristic appearances on x-ray, it is sometimes difficult to tell one from the other just on a single x-ray.

Blood Tests

Blood tests are less subject to misinterpretation. Most tests are compared to a normal range of values for the person's age and sex. Ninety-five percent of people without any abnormality will have blood test results within that so-called normal range. This is like calculating the range of heights of the population. Ninety-five percent of people fall between one lower limit and one upper limit. There are always a few taller or shorter than the average. Even though they fall outside the normal range, they are still normal. So we sometimes find a raised level or low level on a particular blood test, but it does not necessarily mean it is abnormal. However, abnormalities usually occur a long way outside the normal range, and it is not difficult to define whether the test result has been normal or abnormal.

In evaluating rheumatic disease, a blood test helps to detect any *inflammation*. The disease process of inflammation causes changes in the chemical structure of the blood — particularly in protein levels. This in turn can be measured using quick techniques in standard laboratories. The ESR (erythrocyte sedimentation rate) or 'sedrate' is the usual test done to show the presence of inflammation. If the level is up, then the test usually means there is inflammation within the body. However, it doesn't tell you what sort of inflammation or where it is. An elevated sedrate can happen with tonsillitis, appendicitis or arthritis. So, once again, the test has to be considered with the person's complaints and the physical findings.

The next most common test is the full blood examination (or complete blood count): the different parts of the blood are measured. This test shows whether anaemia is present, and may give the cause. It will also show whether the white cells are in the normal range, and whether the platelets (or clotting cells) are normal. A full blood examination often gives lots of information on the general health of the patient.

Other investigations may be used to explain the presence of any underlying arthritis. The *rheumatoid factor* is found in three quarters of people with rheumatoid arthritis. It can also be found in low levels in normal people and after certain infections. So the test does not *prove* the presence of rheumatoid arthritis. It is merely suggestive. The *antinuclear antibody* is a blood test which is also sometimes positive in normal people at low reac-

tion levels. At higher levels it is found in conditions such
as *systemic lupus erythematosus*, a chronic generalised
disorder characterised by inflammation in various
organs such as the joints. Antinuclear antibodies also
occur in rheumatoid arthritis and other conditions.
There are many other investigations that can be performed on the function of the major organs — e.g. on
kidneys, liver, heart, muscle, thyroid glands, or whatever.
These tests may be needed after anyone with a group of
rheumatic symptoms is assessed. In general, though,
only a few tests are necessary before the particular rheumatic condition is named.

8

Rheumatism and Unproven Remedies

At one time or other, every person with rheumatic pain is confronted with a swag of remedies and cures. The remedies may come from neighbours, relatives or friends. 'My aunty had chronic rheumatism until she cut out all meat and changed to non-acid foods.' 'Try that cow manure mixture: it's cured my rheumatic knee.' 'A copper bracelet will do the trick!' You've all heard these stories. Other sources of remedies and cures for rheumatism are newspapers, popular magazines and current affairs TV shows. There's always someone with a new cure ready to tell the world — often for a price!

At one time medicines were sold off the back of a wagon — with their guarantee of longlasting relief for a variety of symptoms, including rheumatism. This word-of-mouth guarantee still persists in the various remedies that circulate through the community. Despite sophisticated knowledge of the human body, the overly simplistic approach between cause and effect still persists even today. Many of the cures for rheumatism are grossly oversimplified 'good ideas' which do not stand up to scientific scrutiny.

Careful Checks and Follow-Ups

Don't let us forget the contribution of scientific method to our understanding of medicine. This approach draws on various ideas that surround any problem. Ideas are easy things to generate. You all get clever ideas about what is causing your aches and pains. However, scientific method takes this a bit further. As a follow-up to a good idea, a theory is generated. The theory tries hard to explain why the idea is a good one. For instance, if rheumatic pain is found to be much less whilst bathing in the sea, you may have the bright idea that salt water helps in the treatment of rheumatism. To explain why salt water is useful, you work out a theory. The theory runs something along these lines: sea water helps my rheumatism, therefore I hypothesise that I lack certain salts which are replaced during bathing in the sea. Most alternative health practitioners generate good ideas and theories to explain these good ideas. However, they may be unable to take the next step that separates them from the orthodox scientific community.

In fact, the crucial next step is to do an experiment: test whether the theory is right. The whole thrust of scientific development has been based on testing whether the hypothesis which comes from a good idea is correct. The hypothesis must be tested by scientific experiment. All hypotheses are capable of being tested. Once the hypothesis has been tested, a result is analysed. If the result indicates that the theory is correct, then the treatment or observation is incorporated into standard medical scientific practice. If it is not proved to be correct, then the hypothesis or theory may be modified and another experiment done to see where the truth lies (Figure 1).

The 'Good Idea'

There are lots of treatments around for rheumatism which are simply good ideas. They may be backed by theories about why they work, but most when scientifically tested fall in a heap.

The same applies to diets for arthritis and rheumatism: most of these too have not been subjected to close scrutiny. A popular diet called Dr Dong's diet has been used for over forty years. It is based on Dr Dong's observations of his own improvement while on the diet. He said, 'It is not a scientific work, in the sense of being based on thorough and well authenticated scientific research.' In 1983 American research workers had a hard look at the Dong diet with a number of volunteers. After ten weeks, they could find no effect of the diet on rheumatic symptoms. So a remedy unproven over forty years, but popularly used due to word of mouth and books, was shown not to work. It would take an incredible amount of research to delve into all the different 'good idea' diets that have been tried.

There is a large clinic in the United States, the Mayo Clinic, to which patients come from all over the country

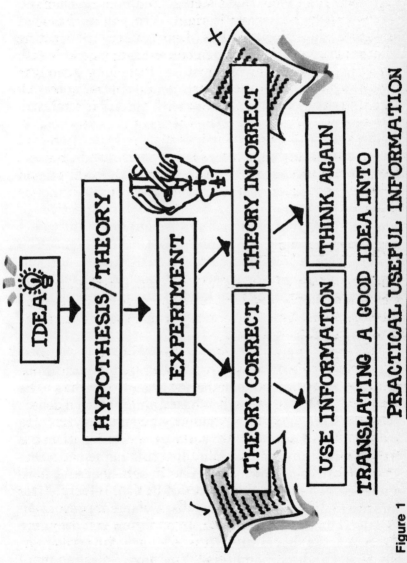

TRANSLATING A GOOD IDEA INTO PRACTICAL USEFUL INFORMATION

Figure 1

seeking advice about rheumatic conditions. One doctor
at the Clinic said that some people claimed to be improving after using the Tomato Diet. He followed this up for a
time, asking whether they had tried the Tomato Diet and
how well it had worked. The interesting thing was that
people coming from one side of the country thought the
Tomato Diet meant they should not eat tomatoes at all,
whilst people from the other side of the country thought
it meant they should eat more tomatoes in their diet. An
equal number of patients from each side of the country
improved on the 'Tomato Diet'. This tells us more about
people than the diet!

Most of those who improve on any one diet do so
because of the 'placebo effect'. This is the well known
effect whereby any treatment will have a 50-50 chance of
causing improvement in symptoms, irrespective of
whether the treatment has any scientific validity. It's
important, though, to have faith in the treatment. You
tend to believe treatments suggested by friends and colleagues and people you trust. Often doctors are regarded
as unhelpful in giving this kind of advice.

Alternative Approaches

Since the late 1970s there has been rapid growth in interest in alternative medicine for lots of disorders. The
growth of alternative medicine is commonest in diseases
of unknown causes — particularly when the symptoms
are troublesome and last for some time. Rheumatism fits
this description to a tee. Why has this happened? One
good reason is a growing interest in self-help and individual responsibility in matters of health. Lifestyle factors are highlighted in causing disease and in prevention
through change in behaviour. In addition, you are more
aware of the harmful effects of medications, drugs,
chemicals and food additives. You have access to more
knowledge. All of these things tend to support the
'simple, traditional and natural' treatments offered by
alternative approaches.

In this context you will find a hierarchy of alternative

medical approaches to rheumatic conditions. Many people use simple things like the copper bracelet, which is quite cheap. Maybe they make a simple change in diet, such as eliminating red meats or changing the balance between 'acid foods' and other foods. Others are more motivated: they opt for a more complicated dietary change, such as the Pritikin diet or one of the other alternatives. Such a change in diet involves more skill and time in choosing foods. You need greater motivation and belief that this complicated diet works.

Yet others use physical treatments for rheumatic complaints — perhaps chiropractic treatment, physiotherapy treatment, hydrotherapy treatment, or other physical approaches. Acupuncture is also used. Of course, care must be taken when considering treatment of rheumatic conditions. Some people make an analogy between the effectiveness of a treatment and the amount of money spent on it.

While there is no doubt that many people have received relief from their rheumatism by one or other of these methods, there are some unscrupulous 'therapists' who can cost you a lot of money without helping your rheumatism.

Some people have tried naturopathic medicine, where attention is focused on the patient's diet and various nutritional supplements may be prescribed, along with treatments such as hydrotherapy.

Others have turned to chelation therapy, where patients are given solutions of chemicals to 'mop up' the chemicals or compounds in their blood which are said to be causing the symptoms. With both of these therapies, again, it is best to choose your practitioner carefully.

The medical profession has its own alternative approaches — for example allergy units where patients can be tested for allergies to foods or chemicals and then desensitised.

None of these treatments has been proved to be useless — if one of them seems to help you, go ahead. But neither have they been scientifically tested. There are many orthodox, proven remedies which *have* been tested.

Claims and Cures

Why then are there so many false claims for cures of rheumatic conditions? There is often an obvious need to do something. It is hard to watch a friend or relative suffering from pain or stiffness or other rheumatic complaint, and not offer help. Most alternative treatments are offered in good spirit, although in some cases there is exploitation of people who will pay for any suggestion of help. It's also exciting to get new ideas and new suggestions about treatments for old conditions. The popular press and current affairs TV programs are full of these 'cures'. Unfortunately the popular press grabs hold of ideas and doesn't wait for scientific testing. Big disappointment then occurs in many people.

Let's go back for a moment to our understanding of rheumatism. You recall that pain from central spinal structures activates pain pathways. These pathways refer pain into the arms or legs or other structures. Other reflex changes occur which produce muscle tightening, circulation changes or other local effects. You also recall that the pain-nerve system is subject to control from central influences. These central influences are poorly understood but do interact with psychological and emotional effects. Psychological events — whether known to the person or not — are of utmost importance in control, modulation or activation of the pain-nerve system. It is at this level that most alternative medical approaches have their effect.

The power of the placebo cannot be underestimated. Alternative medical treatments, diets, physical treatments and the like usually achieve their response through the positive approach of the treater or healer. A simple explanation is offered for the problem, and a solution based on a particular way of treating is suggested. Perhaps the explanation is one of a dietary deficiency, and a new diet is advised. Perhaps there's the suggestion that something is 'out of place' and physical treatment will put that something back in place.

A bag of treatments is used, based on simple-to-understand explanations. These explanations may have nothing to do with the truth, but they serve to focus the patient's mind on a hopeful and positive course. The medium the healer uses is not important: it is the message that is being put across. The moral in this story is the medium does not have to be costly, nor left to someone else. The same positive effects can come from your own efforts. The key point is to remember that psychological and personal factors are far more relevant in rheumatic problems than any others.

Can you remember then how rheumatism is caused? Mostly, it's begun by simple strain or muscle pull in the neck or back. The pain nerve system is excited. Referred pain occurs away from the troublesome spot. Various other reflexes occur, causing muscle tightness, circulation changes and the like.

The control system for all of this resides in the spinal cord. The main regulator of the system comes from central effects on the brain, and of these central effects psychological factors are the most crucial. If you can make the link between psychological factors (whether recognised or unrecognised) and increased pain from simple strains and mechanical problems, then you can do a lot to help yourself. Naturally this approach won't help everyone: a true arthritis may be the root of the problem, or there may be some other tissue damage which won't respond to the psychological modulation you seek. Don't forget that this refers to the simple everyday aches and pains of muscle tension and rheumatism.

Self Healing

You can become your own self-healer without the need for an external powerful person to guide you in your relief of symptoms. Of course many of you will require a powerful external force (e.g. friend, relative, doctor), and you can make a choice from various types of treatment methods. However, most people can achieve the same

effect using their own skills and self-treatment programs.

---

*It is wise to remember that unproven remedies
may have unfortunate effects on health. Such a
case was Maria's. Maria was twenty-five years
old, the mother of three children. She had
systemic lupus erythematosus. It's a chronic
inflammatory disease of unknown cause that
results in inflammation of joints, kidneys, or
other vital internal organs. Maria had a
nine-year history of lupus, well controlled on a
dose of cortisone — a medication which acted as
a powerful anti-inflammatory control for her
condition. She had no side effects from the
medication.*

*Maria went to a naturopath. The advice she
got was to take herbal treatments and stop
cortisone. Eating too many fresh wheat shoots,
coupled with stopping cortisone, led to a severe
flare-up of the lupus, and Maria went to hospital
feeling very ill from inflammation of the kidneys
— a new problem for her. This, in turn, meant
bigger doses of cortisone and a long period of
rehabilitation. Now, she is back to normal health
and on the previous medication. Maria's
experience reminds us that, if you use alternative
approaches, be sure to let your regular doctor
know so both approaches can be incorporated.*

Well, what this chapter advocates is a fresh look at the
use of alternative medicines in rheumatic conditions.
You need, though, to clearly dissect out the vital ingredient in alternative medicine. That vital ingredient is
the positive psychological approach taken by the 'healer'
or alternative medical therapist. The same positive ap-

proach is taken by orthodox medical practitioners and allied health professionals. It is an approach which can also be taken by you as an individual on a day-by-day basis, forming the basis for self-management of difficult disorders.

9

Exercise
and
Rheumatism

Exercise helps most people with rheumatic pain. In its way, it is just as important as relaxation and stress management. In fact exercise is a wonderful way of handling stress. It helps the physical components of pain, as well as complementing mental relaxation to desensitise the pain pathways.

Before you embark on an exercise program, be sure to get a correct diagnosis of your particular type of rheumatism. Simple chronic neck strain with referred pain needs quite different treatment to severe localised fibrositis. Your doctor will help work out the correct diagnosis and map out a plan of management for you. In many situations the diagnosis is clear cut, but there is recurring muscle pain or stiffness. If so, it is a matter of renewing your exercise program if pain or stiffness flares up.

Physical Treatments

Usually it's best to be assessed and get advice from a person skilled in physical therapy. Maybe there is a need for specific treatment for a neck or back complaint before you start off on exercise. The therapist pays particular attention to movements of the low neck and back, or other relevant areas. If these are not very mobile and have stiffened, it may be necessary to loosen up through various techniques. So-called soft tissue mobilisation of the low neck or low back is a common manoeuvre by most physical therapists. They approach this with great care, particularly if you have lots of tender points in the region. It's a situation in which the pain pathways are much activated, and even fairly simple treatments may worsen the pain. If this is the case, heat may be applied for 15 or 20 minutes before treatment. This desensitises the tissues, loosens the muscles, and allows for easier gentle mobilisation to start. If there is local pain, ultrasound or electrical desensitisation (via interferential or transcutaneous nerve stimulation) may be used. The therapist may manage to stretch the tissues beyond their tightened state, and so lessen the central source of pain.

Generally, most of these treatments achieve their

main aims in three of four sessions. They should then be replaced by a self-help exercise program where you take responsibility for your own health care. Too much reliance on therapists leads to dependency — something that is hard to break and is not helpful, especially when there is pain amplification.

In cases of acute flare-ups of pain, you may try ice or heat. A packet of frozen peas from the freezer wrapped in a towel is applied to the sore area for about 20 minutes. Alternatively a hot water bottle wrapped in a towel is applied for a similar period. Some people respond better to ice than to heat. The response is individual. The magic time seems to be 20 minutes for most of these physical treatments, which can be applied at home and repeated when needed. Following application of ice or heat, it's sensible to stretch the area gently — to the point of discomfort but not to the point of pain. This helps to loosen the neck or the back, diminishing the acute episode.

The physical therapist will probably also discuss posture with you. You noted before that posture of the low neck and back is often the focus for pain in those tissues. In the diagram (Figure 1), see poor neck posture. To correct this, do exercises to adopt the posture as shown.

For the low back you can see a similar situation in the diagram (Figure 2). The pelvic tilt is the best to help correct this. See Figure 10 in Chapter 4. Abdominal muscle strengthening exercises also help. Some people find these exercises difficult to do and they can cause back pain. It depends on how bad the problem is, and it's often best to get advice first from your therapist or doctor. Rotation of the low back may also be recommended after your problem is assessed.

In many cases your therapist will recommend that you purchase a good book on exercise routines and then point out the specific ones that are recommended for you. Anyhow, it's difficult to generalise about exercise. In some cases only one exercise may be needed; in others several; and in others perhaps no specific exercise is recommended. In that case what is needed is a general fitness program.

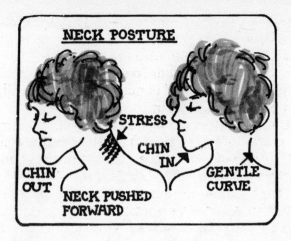

Figure 1

Exercise Is Good for You

After your assessment and advice, you can do lots of the work by yourself at home. It is up to you. Depending on the severity of your problem and your previous level of fitness, there is a number of possibilities.

Walking is a great way to start. You should walk at a brisk pace for up to 20 minutes each day. The aim is to walk for one block on the first day, then increase by another block every day according to your capability. Walking is best in the morning when you are fresh.

Swimming is good exercise too. Again 20-30 minutes a day is a good time span. Gentle side stroke is fine to start with, perhaps followed by a relaxing spa. Some people prefer bicycle riding.

The aim of exercise is to induce stretching and strengthening, relaxation and general fitness. Fitness and relaxation go closely together. As you exercise, your self-confidence and self-esteem will grow. These things are very important when dealing with chronic pain.

A gym is a good place for self help. It's important, however, not to do too much too quickly. Take care when doing activities like aerobics and weight training. You should merge into such programs after you do lots of

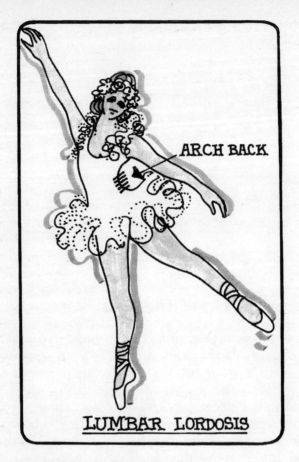

Figure 2

basic walking, swimming or cycling. Be sure to get advice about any gym program you take on.

Many people with chronic pain feel weak in the area of the pain. For instance, if the neck is a source of pain, there may be weakness of the arms, or generalised fibrositis may leave you feeling generally weak. In these situations the muscles are quite normal. They do not waste, and they are able to function quite normally if pain relief occurs. The feeling of weakness is a simple reflex. In other words, muscle tone and strength will improve with pain relief and good posture. There may be no call for specific muscle strengthening exercises, but rather attention to the general principles of relaxation and general exercise.

Movement and Pain

Massage is very helpful. There are many courses now on massage, and massage itself is available from professionals fairly cheaply. There are different types of massage. It's usually best to find one that suits you after trial and error. Try teaching other members of your family to do the massage! That's fun for everyone in the family. In fibrositis, deep massage like shiatsu can aggravate, and often it's wise to start with gentler stretching massage.

There are many other techniques for improving posture, increasing relaxation, and linking body and mind in a natural way. Such techniques as tai chi, Alexander technique, Feldenkrais technique and others are all worth a try. Most people find their own approach, but if you are getting lost and cannot make headway, look at these other techniques that have developed over the years.

Exercise and movement are particularly important in severe localised forms of fibrositis. 'If you don't move it, you lose it' is a very important adage. Despite stiffness and pain, it is crucial to use the arm, the leg, the back or whatever is hurting. Movement decreases pain in the long run. Movement increases your confidence, reassuring you that there is nothing structurally wrong deep inside. Movement is the key to improvement in these situations.

It is not possible for this book to map out an individual set of exercises. There are so many combinations of rheumatic pains that occur with fibrositis, referred pain and other pain syndromes. However, the principles are the important things. Accurate diagnosis, skilled assessment by a person trained in physical therapy, a sensible program and perseverance, especially in the early stages, are all essential.

Finally, don't forget to combine your exercise program with relaxation techniques.

10

Stress
and
Rheumatism
— What To Do

Recognising Stress

If you have chronic rheumatic pain or fibrositis, you should ask yourself the question, 'Am I under stress?' The answer comes from recognising the symptoms of stress.

Stress symptoms may be physical, psychological or social. Figure 1 shows these in diagrammatic form.

● Palpitations, sweating for no apparent reason, fever or high temperature at night, bowel or bladder disturbance without reason, headaches, or just feeling unwell are all physical symptoms of stress. Symptoms in muscles were outlined before: these ranged from mild to severe and came under the heading of fibrositis or one of its variants.

● Psychological symptoms of stress include poor sleep, irritability, trouble with concentration, poor memory, feelings of detachment from the environment, or feelings of impending doom. There are many other psychological symptoms as well.

● Social consequences of stress include excessive use of alcohol or tobacco, becoming withdrawn from friends or acquaintances, and even not going out. Increased sick time from work or just not coping with work may also signal underlying stress. There are many other examples of the features of stress.

At times it needs someone else to point out these stress features to you. Often the suggestion that you are showing signs of stress is not greeted with much enthusiasm. You will deny it for a time. It may take a number of people to point this out, or the passing of time, before you realise that your friends and family are right. Just make sure that, if you are suffering chronic pain or fibrositis, you consider the possibility that stress is in some way involved in the problem.

Once a link between stress and rheumatic symptoms is made, then you have taken a big leap forward. The next step is to identify where the stress arises. Maybe it stems from problems in the family or at work or from other situations. However, the most important person in the stress formula is yourself.

Some Stress Is Normal

A certain amount of stress is normal and always present. It is acceptable, and most of us thrive on some stress. The best performances by top athletes come after incredible stress. Often years of training and mental planning culminate in a single event where the top performance occurs. Well controlled stress promotes students to give their best at examination times. Stage performers 'psyche themselves up' to give of their best. You do that little bit better when under some form of stress. This is healthy. Just as physical stress helps your body tissues develop and flourish, so does emotional stress help your mental health.

At other times you perform badly because you have handled stress poorly. Instead of feeding off the stress and producing better performances, you let the stress get on top and prevent you from doing your best. At times there is a fine line between handling stress well and handling it poorly — a common situation in life. You can liken this to a tennis match. Here you see two highly skilled and physically fit athletes competing in front of a large crowd. The winner of the game is usually the one who handles the stress better, the one who accepts the poor line calls, the one who fights back from a near hopeless position, the one who does not give in. You see a player who is completely in control suddenly crumble when an opponent hits a purple patch. The game can change dramatically by good or bad handling of stress, regardless of the skills of the players. So too in life.

You see people, the most capable and valued members of a family or a community, suddenly change to fearful, unconfident passengers in life. These may be people who manage large businesses with many employees under them; people who stand successfully for public office; people who run busy households and have active social lives. It's always a surprise to discover how the most cap-

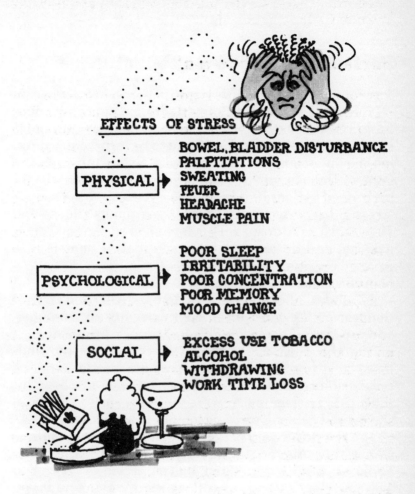

Figure 1

able of people can suddenly 'wobble' and develop severe symptoms of stress. It also amazes how it is often a minor event that is the trigger. This is characteristic of stress reaction. Major stresses such as the death of a spouse or a divorce are often handled fairly well — or so it seems. But a series of lesser stresses produces a more devastating effect on the coping system. Once the symptoms start, a magnifying effect occurs and milder problems just add fuel to the flames.

Perfectionism Can Be Harmful

The important thing with stress is to cope with it properly. How do you avoid changing from a coper to a non-coper? You must be wary. Perfectionists are prone to handling stress poorly. They tend to have difficulty ranking the importance of various tasks. Everything must be done to the best of their ability. If even one task is not performed to their best level, this is a worry. This adds to stress. Such perfectionists show signs of musculoskeletal stress such as fibrositis. They are good workers, keen to perform and do an extremely good job. But it is at a cost.

Perfectionists need to learn to rank the importance of tasks, and to allocate sensible time to tasks and time to themselves. They are often poor delegators of responsibility, particularly in family situations. For example, it may be that the teenage daughter needs the responsibility to make her own decisions in certain matters, and the responsibility should be delegated to her at the right time. Often delegated responsibilities seem small, but in the overall scheme of things small things count.

You should be wary of the 'yes syndrome'. Don't aim to please everyone. Set limits on your activities and limits on how much you can do in a given period of time. You will not offend friends or colleagues by saying no if you cannot cope with some task to the best of your ability. You know this, but it is sometimes hard to admit it. You may feel important if asked to do everything by everyone. For a while you may be able to do it, but again at a cost. The internal awareness of stress often comes too late. It comes after significant symptoms have developed. You will undoubtedly have had symptoms linked to stressful situations, so you must train yourself to recognise stress early.

As well as internal awareness, you must be aware 'externally'. Evaluate external stresses very carefully.

Look at your friends and acquaintances. Stress is catching. If you deal with people 'in the fast lane' and under a lot of stress, you tend to pick up their habits. If you continue in this environment, you should choose some other friends and acquaintances who are not under stress and so balance the emotional equation.

In other words you should both recognise stress and identify ways of coping with that stress. Coping gets back to you as an individual. The final responsibility is yours and not someone else's.

Modifying Stress

● The first thing you need to decide is what your goals are in handling the stress situation. This book deals mainly with rheumatism, the main symptoms of which are pain, stiffness and fatigue. If your goal is to lose all these symptoms totally and forever, then you may be in for a very long battle. If, however, your goal is to minimise the symptoms, then ignore minor complaints, press on and continue life as normally as you can.

● Are your symptoms serious enough to make changes in your lifestyle? The question is important. You do need to examine your priorities. If you have only mild musculoskeletal aches from time to time under obvious stress, then you should not need to make wholesale life changes just for minor discomforts. If, though, you feel that your health — as epitomised by pain, fatigue and stiffness — is suffering because of stress, then you do need to make changes. Ask yourself the question. 'What do I want to be doing in a week or in six months or in twelve months?' If what you want to do depends on few or no symptoms, you know what to work at.

If changes are to be made, recognise that no one activity or change will solve the problem fully. A combination of many things will be needed, some of which are more important than others.

● The single most important ingredient is a positive mental attitude. Approach your health as a winner and not a loser. A positive mental attitude is your single most important weapon against chronic pain. It is normal to have a positive mental attitude, but at times it slips into defeatism and negativism, particularly when you fall into the cycle of chronic pain.

● Good sleep is vital. You'll recollect the scientific and physiological evidence of the link between sleep and fibrositis pain, noting that poor quality sleep was the big problem. It is not the length of sleep that is important. You should aim to have refreshing sleep. You should wake in the morning feeling refreshed. Often excessive sleeping spills over into the day as fuzzy-headedness, drowsiness, irritability and persistence of muscle aching.

Jan was a fifteen-year-old who had severe chest wall pain of the fibrositis type for about two and a half years. She tended to sleep in until 8.30 in the morning. Her problem persisted, fluctuating despite various medications and physical treatments. After advice she began to wake at 6.30 in the morning and do some gentle exercises. After 2–3 weeks the ache in her chest wall began to diminish dramatically. Now, she is coping well, leading an active life like most of her friends.

Try it. If you think you need more sleep and just can't get enough, maybe it's the other way around for you. Maybe you should wake earlier for a few weeks to see if this will break the cycle and increase the quality of sleep. On wakening, do some gentle exercises. This should include a gradual stretch program. If you are aching, stretch slowly and gently. Stretch into the pain and into the joint. Do the stretching before you leave the bed. Tai chi may work for you in encouraging appropriate stretching. Move all the joints and the neck. Move the neck sideways and up and down. Avoid rotating the neck around in a circle. Go for a short walk: with the birds so to speak. Swimming, particularly early in the morning, is also refreshing to mind and body.

To help fall asleep at night, ensure that you go to bed in a relaxed state. Finish all the day's thinking before you enter the bedroom. If problems haven't been solved, put them in the 'dumping basket' of your mind. Come back to them tomorrow. Do not take them into the bedroom and chew on them before you go to sleep or through the night. Make decisions even if the decision is to delay thoughts on any one thing. Remember that sleep is the time between today and tomorrow. It is not today and it is not tomorrow. It is your own time to recuperate bodily strength.

Exercise and Sleep

Sleep comes better after gentle exercise, not vigorous exercise, before bed. Avoid coffee in the hours before bed. Remember that fresh coffee contains 80 mg of caffeine, instant coffee 75 mg and tea 65 mg. Avoid stimulants before going to bed. This includes hot drinks even if they do not contain caffeine. If you have a real sleep problem, cut coffee down to around three cups or less per day. If you have a shower or bath, ensure it is not hot: make it warm. Do not dry yourself vigorously with a towel (this tends to stimulate you), but instead pat yourself dry.

Avoid very hot beds, wear light clothing and use blankets in preference to electric blankets. It is easier to throw off a blanket or quilt in the middle of the night than to change the setting on the electric blanket when you are sweltering. Avoid a cold bedroom too of course.

At times you may need mild medication to modify sleep. This is not to be encouraged, but there are some short-acting mild medications that are useful. A medication like Temazepam may break a poor sleep cycle, decrease nervous system input into painful areas, and help relax muscles. Such a change may stop a flare up of fibrositis or other soft tissue pain. Medications designed for muscle relaxation should not be used as sleep inducers, but be reserved for painful muscle spasm conditions.

Disturbed Sleep

If you have disturbed sleep and there seems to be no help coming from other quarters, the use of tricyclic antidepressant medications is useful. Such medications have been shown scientifically to help patients with fibrositis by levelling out the sleep disturbance. It's felt they encourage a better or deeper sleep. These medications do not act as sleep inducers, so are usually taken around 8 o'clock at night. The maximal effect comes in the early hours of the morning when surfacing from a shallow sleep usually occurs. They are usually given in low doses. They modulate the pain pathways, particularly at the 'relay station' before the pain message heads up to the brain. Even though used in very low doses, they are prone to side effects in people with fibrositis. This probably relates in some way to the reflexes triggered by the fibrositis process. So people may become drowsy in the morning, even after a low dose of this medication. It is important to stick with the medication if your doctor is convinced you need it. It is all too easy to throw away a medication for minor discomfort, and lose a very positive effect on pain that may otherwise last for a long time. If sleep can be improved to give a normal good quality relaxing sleep, then significant improvement in musculoskeletal symptoms usually follows.

Holidays help. Have regular breaks from life's activities. This is why weekends were designed. It is also why most jobs give us breaks through the year, and two weeks holiday every six months is better than four weeks holiday every twelve months. Holidays should be scheduled regularly through the year. Plan them with care.

A holiday with physical activity can be a great relaxation in itself. You feel naturally refreshed on holidays and find that physical activity comes more easily than when you're in the hurly-burly of everyday life. Health resorts and spas are good places for a change. They come in various packages, but it is the message that is important — relax.

People lucky enough to go to spas abroad often send postcards showing beautiful sunny days, inviting pools and spas, and centres which house masseurs and other physical therapists. They talk of the regular physical activity that occurred and their incredible feeling of wellbeing. So plan your holiday and work out the type of holiday that suits your musculoskeletal requirements.

Think About Good Posture

Posture is important. During a medical symposium on pain, an intense rheumatologist lent forward in his chair, his legs and arms crossed and his body hunched over, and asked the speaker 'Can you show me the posture of stress?' The speaker merely said, 'Look at yourself'. As stress increases, you tend to crouch forward, to speak louder, to speak more quickly, to talk in close proximity to people. You hunch your body, lift your shoulders, clench your jaw, furrow your brows, clench your fists, cross your legs and draw yourself up into a tense little ball.

Recognising this posture helps in adopting other postures which induce relaxation in the body throughout the day. For instance, if you sit at your desk or drive your car, you may recognise a strong grip on the wheel or the clenched jaw or the frown. You may lean forward and hunch your shoulders. Merely by recognising this posture, you can correct it. Sit back in the chair, loosen your grip, put a relaxed expression on your face, open your legs rather than hold then closed — all these will induce muscle relaxation and a sense of wellbeing. This is body language at its best. Recognise the body language of stress, and work on a day-to-day basis to minimise it.

Breathing is vital too! Practise the deep sigh. Take a long deep breath every now and then, let it out slowly and let your body relax. Drop the shoulders, sink down into the chair or stand comfortably. Give yourself a few minutes 'breathing space'. You can train yourself to react to a key word such as 'relax' or 'break' or whatever. Say the word slowly under your breath three or four times. Let yourself relax as the word comes to your mind. Practise this regularly. Use the key word as a trigger to relaxation. Remember the most important rule of relaxation. You cannot stop learning and practising relaxation. You must always seek to improve your technique of relaxation. Remember the yogis took twenty or thirty years before they could lie on a bed of nails. You don't need to do that, but you do need to build up skills over months and years.

Another useful technique is to create a visual image of a relaxation retreat. It may be your favourite park bench or a cosy Saturday night fire. It may be somewhere in the country or down on the coast. Create the visual image of this spot in your mind. This is a safe and quiet place for you alone. Bring this image to your mind for thirty seconds or so, let yourself relax, give yourself a respite from the day's activities.

Switch Off Your Tension

Learn to switch off. Imagine a sign with 'stop' on it. As a tense situation arises or stress builds up, visualise the stop sign. Mental and visual imagery can be useful in pain management.

If something is bugging you and you can't quite resolve the problem, write the thoughts down on paper, look at them and resolve the issue. Don't let the thoughts or conflicts nag at you all the time. Most people are capable of making appropriate and usually very good decisions. Be confident. More harm is done by unresolved decisions than by bad decisions.

Rationalisation is useful. Why are you worried? Why worry? Ask yourself, 'How significant will this problem be in five years time?' Try to distance yourself from the problem and use your perspective of life to see exactly how important this little problem is. Look about you;

don't look within yourself. Sure you feel bad but look at others.

One person was cured of fibrositis when she volunteered for a church Meals on Wheels program. During her journeys around the suburbs with the meals for elderly and frail folk, she found many examples of incredible bravery and resolution in people with very significant and serious illnesses. She realised that life wasn't that bad after all. Perhaps her pain, even though it was significant and distressing, should be put aside. There was much in life that she could do and her pain was not going to stop her. She is now coping very well and doing many things that seemed impossible even three months earlier.

Have something to look forward to. Even at the worst times of the day, make sure there is something you enjoy doing that waits you at the end of the day, or sometime in the near future. There is always something enjoyable you can mark down as 'something to look forward to'.

Don't Dwell on Your Pain

With chronic pain, avoid focusing on your problem. It's a major trap. As pain cannot be seen, it is often complained about by one member of the family to others. Yet family relationships do not tolerate this well. Other family members may see the underlying stress or emotional problem more clearly than the person with the pain, yet they may try to distance themselves from the complaints, making cruel and unhelpful remarks. In such situations you can allocate fifteen minutes a day to complain to the family! They can listen, then for the rest of the day the whole problem can be put aside. The pain can be forgotten about. It will still be there, but it is somehow better off for not being discussed. If people stop you in the street and ask you how you are, say 'I am fine'. Don't start to tell them about your pain. You will look good. People with chronic pain usually do. There is not much to show for itself. The more you act normally, talk normally and communicate normally, the less important the pain will be.

In some families a special relationship occurs between the person with the pain and the spouse, son or daughter — or with an outsider. This person acts as a nurturing individual. He or she feels lots of empathy with the person with the pain. He or she accompanies the person with the pain everywhere, helps them to dress or eat or get into cars, and generally overviews life. Such a nurturing individual in fact plays into the hands of the sufferer of chronic pain. Even though this is kindness at its extreme, it is not wise. The patient with chronic pain has to learn to be independent, to handle the problem, and to cope with life without props from other people. This is not to say that you should not show compassion and empathy for people with chronic pain. Of course you should. But if you give too much, you risk making the situation worse. It's a delicate situation and may need skilled advice in handling it. Remember that mollycoddled children often fail to develop to fully mature people. Sometimes you have to be 'cruel to be kind' in helping people confront and then deal with chronic pain.

Stress Is Very Personal

Throughout this chapter you have read a lot about stress — ways it presents and ways you can modify it. When stress results in physical symptoms, some people talk about the condition as psychosomatic. The term is used less nowadays. This does not mean that the symptoms are not real. Indeed we have gone to great lengths to explain how real the symptoms are, but you must appreciate the link between psychological stress factors and the resultant symptoms.

If the symptoms cause a change in function of the body tissues without any change in the structure, it is called a functional disorder. Again, the symptoms are very real. However, some may use the term 'functional' to classify or describe the symptoms. This is not to say that the symptoms are imaginary or the person is malingering;

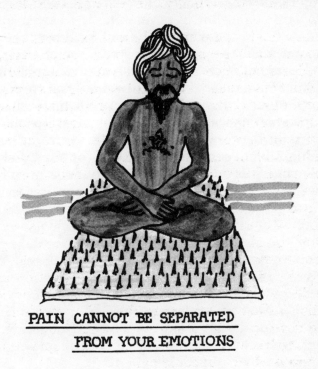

PAIN CANNOT BE SEPARATED
FROM YOUR EMOTIONS

nor is it to say the patient is hysterical or neurotic. Unfortunately, for too long, the medical profession has used these words in a loose manner. This has created many problems which now need re-education throughout the community.

In closing, let's make just a few further points. The first is to remind you that stress is a very personal problem. The problem lies within the person with the symptom. The solution comes from the person with the problem, not from a magic external source. Outside people can help a lot, but they cannot give the magic ingredient. That ingredient lies within you: it just needs to be used properly. Secondly, the suggestions and ideas above are not an exhaustive list of possibilities for stress management. They won't help everyone with stress. They cover just some of the ground, some of the areas that can be tackled. These are quite different from other routine treatments. It may help you to seek the help of a skilled pain counsellor in developing the best program for yourself. This person may be a clinical psychologist, an occupational therapist, a doctor or another highly trained person. Such a person should be trained and skilled in pain management. At times, too, severe depression and other true psychological problems occur that need specific medical treatment. For most people with chronic pain, depression is not a major feature, as long as the pain problem can be handled; but for a few a skilled expert in psychiatric help is needed. Your doctor will help you decide if this is best.

Good Reading

Jayson, M. and Dixon, A., *Rheumatism and Arthritis*, rev. ed., Pan Books, 1984

McKenzie, R., *Treat Your Own Back*, Spinal Publications, 1983.

McKenzie, R., *Treat Your Own Neck*, Spinal Publications, 1983.

Newman Turner, R., *Banish Back Pain*, Thorsons, 1989.

Peck, C., *Controlling Chronic Pain: a Self-Help Guide*, Fontana/Collins, 1982.

Sayce, V., and Fraser, I., *Exercise Beats Arthritis*, Thorsons, 1988.

References

Gowers, W. R., Lumbago: Its Lesions and Analogues, *British Medical Journal*, 1904, 1: 117–121

Moldofsky, H., Scarisbrick, P., England, R., Smythe, H. A., Musculoskeletal Symptoms and Non-REM Sleep Disturbance in Patients with Fibrositis Syndrome and Healthy Subjects, *Psychosomatic Medicine*, 1975, 37: 341–357.

Smythe, H. A., Fibrositis as a Disorder of Pain Modulation, *Clinical Rheumatic Diseases*, 1979: 823–832.

Smythe, H. A., Fibrositis and Other Musculoskeletal Syndromes. In Kelly, W. N., et al (eds), *Textbook of Rheumatology*, W. B. Saunders, 1985, 481–489.

Useful Addresses

Arthritis and Rheumatism Council
41 Eagle Street, London WC1R 4AR. Tel: 071 405 8572

Arthritis Care
6 Grosvenor Cresent, London SW1X 7ER.
Tel: 071 235 0902

National Back Pain Association
31-33 Park Road, Teddington, Middlesex TW11 0AB.
Tel: 081 977 5474

Scoliosis Association
380-384 Harrow Road, London W9. Tel: 071 289 5652

Arthritis Foundation
1314 Spring Street NW, Atlanta, Georgia 30309, USA

Glossary

Acute: Of short duration. This term does not relate to severity, just the length of time.

Analgesics: Medications which act to decrease pain only.

Anti-inflammatory medications: Medications which control inflammation. In doing so, they help ease the pain caused by inflammation, but they may also independently act as pain relievers in their own right.

Arthritis: Disease, damage or abnormality in a joint. There are over one hundred different types, all with different effects.

Bursa: Sac of fluid separating tissues that need to move over each other.

Capsule: Outer lining of joints.

Cartilage: Soft tissue situated at the ends of bones within joints.

CT Scan, Computed Tomography: X-ray which uses computer help to show slices of tissue, including bones, ligaments, nerves, muscles and discs.

Chronic: Long lasting. This term does not relate to severity, just the length of time.

Degeneration: Process by which the structure of an organ (e.g. a joint) breaks down.

Dermatographia: Red reaction seen on the skin after light stroking.

Disc: Structure which separates the bones of the spine. Discs have a spongy soft centre and strong outer fibres, which can at times stretch, strain or rupture — letting the inner disc material ooze out and irritate nerves.

Dislocation: Complete movement of two sides of a joint out of alignment.

Enthesis: Means 'insert into'; the region where tendons or ligaments attach to bone. A most important region, prone to much trauma.

Facet joint: Special type of joint in the back that allows movement.

Fibromyalgia: Literally meaning pain and aching in muscle and fibrous tissue, this term is synonymous with fibrositis.

Fibrositis: Term to define a special type of rheumatism where there is a typical pattern of aches, pains, tenderness and other features. The use of this term implies that no other cause for the symptoms is present.

Hyperostosis: Increased bone.

Hypertrophy: Enlargement.

Inflammation: Process by whichs the body responds to injury, insult or illness; it can affect any organ including joints. Inflammation involves change in blood flow, appearance of special blood cells and, later, healing. The special inflammatory blood cells can produce proteins that cause fever, fatigue and other effects.

Interferential: Type of therapy to deliver heat to deep tissues.

Ligament: Strong band of fibrous tissue which controls excessive movement, particularly around joints.

Lumbago: Dull pain in the low back of any cause.

Manipulation: Forceful movement of a joint beyond its

usual normal range. Designed to stretch surrounding tissues and allow resumption of normal joint movements.

Mechanoreceptors: Nerves which tell you how much stretch or strain is taking place in a joint, muscle or other movable structure.

Mobilisation: Gentle stretching of a joint to loosen surrounding stiffness; performed within the usual normal range of joint motion.

Musculoskeletal system: General term to describe all the components of the body which allow you to move, bend, lift and do things. This includes muscles, ligaments, tendons, joints, bones and many other structures.

Myalgia: Muscle aches or pains.

Myalgic encephalomyelitis: Term applied to combination of severe fatigue, general aching, headache and memory disturbance. Thought to be due to a hidden viral cause, this term is overused and not specific. Many people with this diagnosis have simple good old fibrositis.

Myelogram: X-ray which requires dye to be instilled into the spinal nerve space; this allows the course of the nerves to be outlined.

Narcotic: Type of pain-relieving medication with addictive properties, which is never indicated for chronic pain due to rheumatism, fibrositis, arthritis or any other musculoskeletal diseases.

Osteoarthritis: Special type of arthritis where the cartilage breaks down, followed by bony spurs and joint fluid. The common arthritis as you age.

Osteophyte: Bony spur in an osteoarthritic joint.

Psychological: Term used to encompass all events and processes that occur in the mind: stress events, sleep, worries, ideas, perceptions, coping, relationships, feelings, mood, and many more.

Psychosomatic: Term which relates a physical change in the body ('soma') to a psychological stress phenomenon (e.g. an ulcer due to stress).

Referred pain: Pain starting in a structure deep in the body will cause pain to be felt at some distance away and on the body's surface.

Rheumatism: General term to describe aches and pains not immediately attributable to a known cause.

Scheuermann's disease: Change in development of the spine during the teen years, it occurs in about one person in five and usually does not have any symptoms. It is caused by the disc bulging into the vertebral bodies, above or below.

Sciatica: Pain caused by irritation of the large sciatic nerve in the low back, with pain radiating to the leg. *Often wrongly used* to mean any pain in the back that radiates into the leg.

Scoliosis: Abnormal sideways curve of the spine, usually mild and causing no symptoms.

Spina bifida occulta: One of a number of changes in the development of the spine which occurs in 20 percent of the population and which occasionally has severe symptoms.

Spondylolisthesis: Abnormal movement of one vertebra over another; usually associated with degeneration of the spine.

Spondylosis: Degeneration of the discs or joints of the spine.

Stenosis: Narrowing (e.g. of area where the nerves leave the bony canal in the neck — a 'pinched nerve'!).

Subluxation: Partial movement of the two sides of a joint out of alignment.

Substance P: One of a number of small hormones thought to be important in relaying pain messages.

Syndrome: Collection of symptoms and signs which make a specific and reproducible pattern. Not used where the *cause* of the symptoms and signs is known.

Synovium: Lining of joints, tendon sheaths and bursae, it provides fluid for nutrition and lubrication. Prone to inflammation in many types of arthritis or after injury or with degeneration.

Tender points: Areas of increased tenderness — compared to surrounding areas — located in predictable spots; particularly common in the low neck, chest wall and low back.

Tendon: Structure linking muscles to the part of the body that needs to be moved.

Tenosynovium: Lining of tendon sheaths, especially where they run over flexible or rough areas of the body (e.g. wrist).

Torticollis: Medical term to describe sudden severe neck pain with muscle tightness.

Transcutaneous nerve stimulation: Electrical stimulation of the skin, designed to block out feeling from pain nerves.

Tricyclics: Medications which in high dose act as antidepressants, but which in low dose may improve sleep quality or reduce pain.

Trigger point: Abnormal area which may develop in a muscle which is exquisitely tender. Pressing on a trigger point will greatly increase the pain that was the original complaint.

Ultrasound: Type of therapy to deliver heat to deep tissues.

Index

Of further interest:

A Doctor's Proven New Home Cure for Arthritis

Giraud W. Campbell, D.O. in association with Robert B. Stone

Giraud W. Campbell describes his radical seven day programme which gives relief from osteo and rheumatoid arthritis.

This drugless home remedy is based upon dietary change. Processed foods, caffeine and alcohol are removed and are replaced by basic natural foods such as fruit, vegetables, fish and dairy products.

The method details recipes to follow up the seven day programme, to regain the normal use of limbs and ensure an arthritis-free life.

Giraud W. Campbell has helped hundreds of arthritis sufferers return to normal healthy lives with his natural methods. This cure is so simple that it has been largely ignored until now.

ISBN 0 7225 1911